THE CANCER CURE THAT WORKED!

FIFTY YEARS OF SUPPRESSION

Written by
BARRY LYNES

First printing March 1987
Second printing January 1989
Third printing August 1989
Fourth printing April 1992
Fifth printing August 1994
Sixth printing October 1997
Seventh printing June 1999
Eighth printing August 2000
Ninth printing November 2001

Published in Canada by Marcus Books,
P.O.Box 327, Queensville, Ontario,
Canada L0G 1R0. (905) 478-2201
Fax (905) 478-8338

Cover designed by Doris Diehl

ISBN 0-919951-30-9

The health of the people is really the foundation upon which all their happiness and all their powers as a State depend.

Benjamin Disraeli

Truth will come to light; murder cannot be hid.

Shakespeare

CONTENTS

The People Who Made This Book

Royal R. Rife, born in 1888, was one of the greatest scientific geniuses of the 20th century. He began researching a cure for cancer in 1920, and by 1932 he had isolated the cancer virus. He learned how to destroy it in laboratory cultures and went on to cure cancer in animals. In 1934, he opened a clinic which successfully cured 16 of 16 cases within three months time. Working with some of the most respected researchers in America along with leading doctors from Southern California, he electronically destroyed the cancer virus in patients, allowing their own immune systems to restore health. A Special Research Committee of the University of Southern California oversaw the laboratory research and the experimental treatments until the end of the 1930s. Follow-up clinics conducted in 1935, 1936 and 1937 by the head of the U.S.C. Medical Committee verified the results of the 1934 clinic. Independent physicians utilizing the equipment successfully treated as many as 40 people per day during these years. In addition to curing cancer and other deadly diseases, degenerative conditions such as cataracts were reversed. Rife had been able to determine the precise electrical frequency which destroyed individual micro-organisms responsible for cancer, herpes, tuberculosis, and other illnesses. His work was described in *Science* magazine, medical journals, and later the Smithsonian Institution's annual report.

Unfortunately, Rife's scientific theories and method of treatment conflicted with orthodox views. His work was stopped and both the research and the treatments were forced underground. Doctors secretly continued curing cancer patients for 22 years after the original success of the 1934

1

clinic, but always with opposition from medical and governmental authorities. However, from 1950 to the mid-1980s, a number of research scientists, working independently, have slowly been verifying the scientific principles upon which Rife's clinical cures of the 1930s were based. A body of recognized scientific evidence now overwhelmingly supports the original cancer theories articulated and demonstrated by Rife 50 years ago. This includes modern AIDS researchers.

In the 1950s, *John Crane*—engineer, machinist, laboratory analyst, health researcher and inventor—became Rife's partner. Crane, born in 1915, worked at Rife's side from 1950 until Rife's death in 1971. During this time, he learned all the secrets of Rife's cancer cure . . . and all the details of its suppression. Together, the two men designed and constructed new and better equipment, and managed to interest a new generation of doctors in the possibilities of a genuine, lasting and painless cancer cure. And again the authorities struck. Crane was jailed, equipment was smashed, records were destroyed. Again the motives driving on the forces of suppression were the same. By sharing the long hidden facts, as well as thousands of documents preserved from the 1930s, Crane has enabled the full story to be told.

Author *Barry Lynes*, born in 1942, is an investigative reporter who lives in California. His areas of research, articles and books include economic theory, climate changes, history, U.S.-Soviet relations and alternative health treatments. In early 1986, he became acquainted with John Crane and heard the 'entire Rife story first-hand. Initially skeptical, Lynes changed his mind after examining the wealth of documents in Crane's possession. Outraged by the injustices that had destroyed Rife's work, Lynes decided to reveal in book form what had happened.

You hold the result in your hands.

Foreword

Quantum theory has shown the impossibility of separating the observer from the observed. Proponents of the classical scientific method find this a bitter pill, and little or nothing has been done in a practical way to apply this phenomenon in the everyday practice of science.

This state of affairs is perhaps not surprising. The practice of science continues to be plagued by an oversimplified model of human sight-perception. Much scientific controversy, as well as ongoing prejudice against new discoveries, can be traced to the false assumption that sight follows some uniform law of nature. In fact, *diversity* is the natural law of human sight, an example of diversity within species. This law cannot be changed. However, it can be understood, and its properties defined with sufficient clarity and emphasis to vastly improve both the interpretation of perceptions and the exercise of ethical practices in scientific research.

From individual to individual all of the five senses are *quantitatively* unequal. For example, some of us cannot see without eye glasses, or hear without a hearing aid, taste subtle flavors, smell a rose or feel fine textures. Further, the *quality* of the senses varies with the nature of acquired knowledge or experience of the individual. Relatively, sight contributes more than any of the other senses to our awareness of the world, our being, our consciousness. The eye-mind circuit is itself a variable. A psychologist, studying brain-damaged individuals found a man who thought his wife was a hat. Are there subclinical cases of this phenomenon among us, even scientists? Strangely, this capricious sense is so much a part of most of us we pay it little heed. Who among us can say with certainty

3

they have not played the role of the native in the following script from Magellan's logbook.

"When Magellan's expeditions first landed at Terra del Fuego, the Fuegans, who for centuries had been isolated with their canoe culture, were unable to *see* the ships anchored in the bay. The big ships were so far beyond their experience that, despite their bulk, the horizon continued unbroken: The ships were invisible. This was learned on later expeditions to the area when the Fuegans described how, according to one account, the shaman had first brought to the villagers' attention that the strangers had arrived *in* something which although preposterous beyond belief, could actually be *seen* if one looked carefully. We ask how could they not see the ships . . . they were so obvious, so *real* . . . yet others would ask how *we* cannot see things just as obvious."

Nowhere is the frailty of sight-perception so troublesome as in microscopy. Recently, a medical writer stated that 100 years ago the microscope was a mysterious instrument. No doubt it was at that time, but today it is an even more mysterious instrument. Tools and techniques of essentially infinite variety have evolved to extend human vision enormously, but with inherent complexities. The microscope itself contains the variables of lens configuration, magnification, resolution and lighting. Thousands of stains and staining techniques, evolved over many years, have contributed heavily to complexifying the art of microscopy. While microscopists acknowledge these inherent variables, in uncharted waters they remain extremely troublesome.

But the microscope does more than simply magnify small objects to visible size, it transports the mind's eye into a world of incredible complexity of form, flux and process, especially when the specimen is alive or was once alive. The space traveler has access to better means of orientation than does the microbiologist.

Thus, the microscope is at once a marvelous tool and a reservoir of seemingly endless confusion even without introducing the factor of variations in human sight-perception. No doubt, we should stand in awe of progress made. But we cannot longer thus stand. Old health problems have become more serious, and new ones appear almost daily. Royal Raymond Rife's story contains crucial information to be brought into focus through correlations with both old and new knowledge.

A number of events in the history of microscopy and microbiology lend credence to Rife's discoveries and insights into the nature of his travails.

Circa 1870, Antoine Bechamp saw tiny motile bodies with his microscope which he named "microzymas." In the first third of the 20th century Gunther Enderlein saw these bodies and called them "endobionts." Wilhelm Reich, in the late 1930s, saw a similar if not identical body which he named "bion." There were others during this era. Today in Sweden and in Canada the properties of these same living particles are being explored by researchers who have assigned names from their own imaginations. The various theories advanced by members of this group of researchers remain rejected or largely forgotten. Remarkably, *they all used dark-field condensers,* a known but *uncommon practice.* In microbiology it is particularly difficult to convince others of the truth and value of discoveries made with uncommon methods of observation.

Rife employed a system of lighting as unknown to microscopy today as it was in the 1930s. It was not simply *uncommon,* it was *unknown.* This was the first and most fundamental technical strike against understanding Rife's microscope and biological discoveries. Fear of the unknown is greater than fear of the unfamiliar. Even scientists are not immune to this human instinct.

There were a few who were not distracted by Rife's unknown method of lighting. Having a look at his work, they jumped to the next problem, that of their own dogma, which said it is simply impossible to realize such high magnifications and resolutions with a light microscope, and therefore we do not believe what we see. You, Mr. Rife, are dishonest, and for trying to pull the wool over our eyes we will put troublesome clouds in your skies to the end of your days. Dogma is necessary, but it often lives too long, and is too often exercised unwisely.

Only recently have discoveries been confirmed in biophysics to make it possible to understand the principle by which Rife's microscopes produced magnifications and resolutions so far beyond the limits of conventional light microscopes. Remarkably, the basic phenomena behind these "new" discoveries were described by Gustav Le Bon, psychologist turned physicist, just before the turn of the Century. Then as now, gifted individuals who cross disciplinary boundaries are not heard.

Biophysicists have now shown that there exists a crucial natural interaction between living matter and photons. This process is measurable at the cellular (bacterium) level. Other research has demonstrated that living systems are extraordinarily sensitive to extremely low-energy electromagnetic waves. This is to say, each kind of cell or microorganism has a specific frequency of interaction with the electromagnetic spectrum. By various means, Rife's system allowed adjusting the frequency of light impinging on the specimen. By some insight he learned that the light frequency could be "tuned" into the natural frequency of the microorganism being examined to cause a resonance or feed-back loop. In effect, under this condition, it can be said the microorganism illuminated itself.

Is it possible the newly discovered electromagnetic properties of living matter were visible to certain highly skilled microscopists with nothing more special than a gifted sense of sight? In self defense, Wilhelm Reich, who could see with his microscope what others could not, said a good microscopist must learn to resonate with the specimen. Barbara McClintock, Nobel Prize winning corn geneticist, who experienced years of travail because she could see the un-seeable, explained that she "had a feeling for the organism". Perhaps Rife had such a gift of sight or insight as these two, but he applied it to building a device he hoped would make it possible for all to see further into the mysteries of living things. His device worked, but the world remained blind to these mysteries.

Rife extrapolated from his lighting technique, which we may be certain *he* understood, that specific electromagnetic frequencies would have a negative effect on specific bacterial

6

forms. There can remain no doubt that Rife demonstrated the correctness of his hypothesis to himself and those few who had the courage to look and the perceptual acuity to *see*! The same new discoveries in biophysics not only explain Rife's principle of illumination, they also explain his process for selective destruction of bacteria. The latter phenomenon is similar to ultra-sonic cleaning, differing in delicate selectivity of wave form and frequency. Recently, researchers whose findings have been suppressed, have *caused and cured* cancer in the same group of mice by subjecting them to certain electromagnetic fields. Rife's work was far more sophisticated. He selected specific microscopic targets, and actually *saw* the targets explode.

Rife's works demonstrated beyond a shadow of a doubt that bacteria are pleomorphic rather than monomorphic. This demonstration did more to bring down upon him the wrath of the worst kind of politics of science than any other facet of his work. It violated the strongest of established biological dogmas, that of the germ theory of disease . . . specific etiology. Everyone *knew* this-that-and-the-other disease was *caused* by a characteristic germ. This had been absolutely proven by Koch's postulates and the success of vaccinations.

No one remembered Antoine Bechamp's microzyma theory which said that various conditions of disease evoke the appearance of characteristic bacterial forms from tiny living prebacterial particles which he found in all living systems, and in inert organic matter which had once been alive. This required that bacteria be pleomorphic, a fact he extensively demonstrated, but not to the satisfaction of those who ran the politics of science during the late 1800s. In Bechamp's theory, bacteria are a *symptom* rather than the final *cause* of disease. Today's biologists find these concepts incomprehensible even though both bacterial pleomorphism and endogenous sources of bacteria have been demonstrated repeatedly since Bechamp's time. Perhaps the continuing failure to control both old and new diseases will pressure medical science into realizing that the traditional germ theory dogma is at best incomplete.

During the late 1800s the future course of medical bacteriol-

7

ogy was set largely by expediency. The scientists had *some* answers concerning infectious diseases, and it made good political and commercial sense to put these answers into practice. Bechamp's ideas were not only strange and distasteful, they were complicated. In fact, Bechamp's theory probably relates more to degenerative diseases than to infectious diseases, the latter being of greater concern in that era.

Vaccinations worked, though their real efficacy and long-term effects are now being questioned. The germ theory itself was relatively obvious, and it was easy to convince the public that the cause of their ills was a *thing,* which though invisible, came from outside the body. This gave the individual a distance from the "cause". Though small, this distance was comforting in an era when the nature of disease was so mysterious. The germ theory was embraced with a great sigh of relief; it was ever so much better than nothing. Try as they might, Rife and his highly competent affiliates could not change the color of this dogma.

Today, the fact of bacterial pleomorphism is recognized quietly by small groups of microbiologists who acknowledge not knowing for certain what to do about it. The fact stands without theory, together with other self-evident biological phenomena such as evolution and symbiosis. The processes of pleomorphism appear complex beyond comprehension. It is a *process* rather than a *thing*. Understanding this process has been hampered by the fact that microbiologists have rarely looked at living specimens. Preoccupied with stains and staining techniques, and entranced by the electron microscope, they have continued to look at killed specimens. There is little doubt that Rife's live-specimen microscopy confused his critics, adding strength to their antagonism, and to their conviction they had *not* witnessed bacterial pleomorphism.

Understanding bacterial pleomorphism in a practical way is necessary to unraveling the mysteries of the immune system and degenerative diseases. If one steps outside traditional microbiology, and can somehow insulate oneself from all the controversy and tragic-ridden hindsight, perhaps new light can be brought to the subject. Pleomorphism means simply, "the assumption of various distinct forms by a single organism or species; also the property of crystallizing in two or more forms". (Dorland's Illustrated Medical Dictionary.): or: "1. *Bot.* the occurrence of two or more forms in one life cycle. 2. *Zool.* same as polymorphism" (Webster).

In both the long run and the short run, life is pleomorphic. What do we mean by the long run? There is now convincing evidence that life existed on Earth at least 3,400 million years ago. If life itself on Earth were extinguished today, it would have experienced an enormously long life cycle during which it changed from isolated single cells into an infinite variety of complex living forms. In this sense of the infinity of life, life is pleomorphic. We experience the short run, the periodic forms of living things which collectively perpetuate the infinity of the whole of life itself. The periodic forms we commonly perceive—plants, animals, birds, bees—are obviously pleomorphic . . . in the short run, i.e., minutes, hours, days, weeks, months, years, decades, centuries.

All sexually reproducing life forms begin as a group of identical cells which differentiate into specialized cells which by symbiotic associations create complex living forms such as the human animal. Between fertile egg and birth, the embryo has many forms. The mature animal is a "form of forms."

Even the human intellect may be said to be pleomorphic. Education and experience change its "form," if you will allow this concept. In the English language there is the word *tautology*, meaning: "needless repetition of an idea in a different word, phrase or sentence, redundancy; pleonasm." In the meaning of this word is there not evidence of an instinctive need to somehow change *form?*

Pleomorphism is a self-evident-facts-without-theory property of living systems of the same class as, for example, symbiosis and evolution. Bacteria are living things. They cannot be other than pleomorphic, symbiotic and evolutionary.

Only during the past few years has an interest in live-specimen microscopy emerged together with an assortment of improved light microscopes. These new scopes employ innovative light-paths alone or together with ultraviolet or near-ultraviolet light sources. Ultraviolet light has a strong negative effect on practically all bacteria. In desperation, this compromise is perhaps being too eagerly accepted. Many of the new scopes employ image-enhancement by computer, a technique which may or may not encourage agreement in microbiological perceptions. It may introduce greater complexities than has staining. The bottom line, of course, is that microbiologists must create a whole living-specimen-paradigm within which they can get their heads together. An enormous learning period looms ahead, complicated by tools of ever increasing intricacy.

In retrospect, Rife's microscope appears relatively simple and straightforward, ideally suited for observing living specimens. None of the new light scopes can begin to approach the magnification and resolution achieved by Rife. Only one, a little-known instrument developed in France during the 1960s, approximates that of Rife. Today, this microscope is being operated at 4500 magnifications with an unbelievable 150 angstrom resolution. It *appears* to be an ordinary high-quality research instrument fitted with a dark-field condenser and a light source comprised of a mix of near-ultraviolet and laser, both being of an undisclosed frequency. Its principle of operation may approximate Rife's in a limited way.

A personal note: With my own eyes and with my own research-grade microscope, fitted with a dark-field condenser, I have seen a bacterial pleomorphic process in fresh untreated specimens of human blood. I could not have "seen" this if I had not "known" what to look for. I knew what to look for because I had studied Bechamp, Rife, Reich and others, *and* because of the personal tutorage of a gifted microscopist who had studied the phenomenon for over twenty-five years.

Barry Lynes makes a strong case for replicating Rife's works, his microscope, and especially the electromagnetic frequency generator that Rife's associates used successfully in the clinical treatment of cancer. This would be highly desirable. Rife's works should, by all means, be reexamined *fairly* in light of "new" knowledge. This "new" knowledge has defined, but not answered, many questions. The products of Rife's gentle genius were premature, and they may well contain crucial clues or whole answers.

John W. Mattingly
Colorado State University

THE CANCER CURE THAT WORKED!

AUTHOR'S WARNING

Important. Throughout this book, bacteria and viruses may seem to be confused. Part of the difficulty is based on the simple fact that in 1990s scientific language, viruses are basically defined as extraordinarily small microbes consisting of DNA or RNA (the gene-carrying nucleic acids) surrounded by a coat of protein, and requring a living cell to reproduce. Bacteria are much larger, living microbes consisting of a single cell which reproduces through division.

In the 1930s, bacteria which passed through tiny filters were called "filterable viruses." Later the term filterable was dropped. The "filterable bacteria" which Rife identified as a cause of cancer and which he later called a virus *remains in the 1990s an essentially unexamined area of science.*

If this is still confusing, read chapter 18 <u>first</u>, keeping in mind that most of this book was written hurriedly in October 1986 in just three weeks, and remarkably published quickly and heroically in April 1987 by a courageous publisher. Mainstream American publishers were still afraid to touch the "Rife topic" in 1996! Also keep in mind that it is "energy medicine" or "resonance healing" that is curing many disease conditions, including cancer, just 10 years after this book's original publication, in 1997. The technology and discoveries are exploding as I write this, despite an old guard medical, scientific and government elite that are working furiously to keep the new healing instruments away from the public and beyond any media/public debate.

Chapter 1
The Cure For Cancer

In the summer of 1934 in California, under the auspices of the University of Southern California, a group of leading American bacteriologists and doctors conducted the first successful cancer clinic. The results showed that cancer was caused by a micro-organism, that the micro-organism could be painlessly destroyed in terminally ill cancer patients, and that the effects of the disease could be reversed.

The technical discovery leading to the cancer cure had been described in *Science* magazine in 1931. In the decade following the 1934 clinical success, the technology and the subsequent, successful treatment of cancer patients was discussed at medical conferences, disseminated in a medical journal, cautiously but professionally reported in a major newspaper, and technically explained in an annual report published by the Smithsonian Institution.

However, the cancer cure threatened a number of scientists, physicians, and financial interests. A cover-up was initiated. Physicians using the new technology were coerced into abandoning it. The author of the Smithsonian article was followed and then was shot at while driving his car. He never wrote about the subject again. All reports describing the cure were censored by the head of the AMA (American Medical Association) from the major medical journals. Objective scientific evaluation by government laboratories was prevented. And renowned researchers who supported the technology and its new scientific principles in bacteriology were scorned, ridiculed, and called liars to their face. Eventually, a long, dark silence lasting decades fell over the cancer cure. In time, the cure was labeled a "myth"—it never happened. However, documents now available prove that the cure did exist, was

13

tested successfully in clinical trials, and in fact was used secretly for years afterwards—continuing to cure cancer as well as other diseases.

Yet, despite the blackout which prevented doctors and researchers from knowing about and improving the cure, other scientific investigators continued to verify the basic principles. In the late 1940s and early 1950s, cooperating researchers at a hospital laboratory in New Jersey and a research institute in Pennsylvania made similar discoveries which unknowingly aligned them with the California group of a decade earlier. In 1950, these researchers prepared to make a presentation before the New York Academy of Sciences. But again, political forces intervened and the symposium was cancelled.

Then, in 1953, the basic science which validated the theories of the California group was explained by the New Jersey group at an international microbiology conference in Rome, Italy. The New York Times and the Washington Post reported the discovery.

However, upon the group's return to America, they discovered that the same powerful forces which had prevented an American announcement in 1950 had secretly managed to terminate the financing of the New Jersey laboratory. The leading researcher was forced to move to California and start anew.

In December of that same year, the leader of the California group and the man most responsible for the successful healing of cancer in the 1930s—after years of silence—published a description of the methods and results of the cancer cure. The authorities at the government's National Cancer Institute in Washington, D.C. received a copy at the National Library of Medicine outside Washington, D.C. in Bethesda, Maryland. But they ignored it. The library staff responsible for filing and circulating such reports to the officials determining cancer research policy either failed to do their jobs or they met with opposition from those in charge of the war on cancer.

Still, new researchers continued to appear on the scene. The process of rediscovering what the California group had found continued. In the late 1950s, an international conference was held in Europe. The topic was the same topic which the

California group had championed in the 1930s and which played a critical part in their successful cancer cure.

In 1959, another cancer researcher tested the cancer micro-organism on herself! And developed cancer. But again, the event had little impact in the scientific hierarchy which managed the cancer program.

Finally, in 1967, the work of the Pennsylvania group was reported in the Annals of the New York Academy of Sciences.

Then, in 1969, the New Jersey group presented its findings to the New York Academy of Sciences and requests for reprints poured in from around the country. Yet the cancer authorities—determining how public and private research (and treatment) would be funded—again ignored the discoveries which now were scientific, laboratory-replicable facts.

In 1974, a major work in the bacteriology field was published. It showed how the claims of the bacteriologists involved in the 1930s California clinic had been validated in the ensuing decades. Laboratory proof after laboratory proof convincingly demonstrated that the orthodox theories of the cancer authorities who dominated virus and bacteria research as well as cancer treatment in the 1930s, 1940s, 1950s and 1960s were fundamentally wrong.

In 1976, the first article in 30 years describing the California group's technology and clinical results was published in a popular magazine. The article appeared in *New Age Journal* from Boston, Massachusetts. It outlined 40 years of inattention and suppression by the cancer authorities. At that time, the magazine had a small circulation although it is now nationally distributed monthly. But again, nothing happened. Neither the public nor the medical professionals pursued the medical story of the 20th century—a tested, verified, painless cure for cancer.

In 1980, two French researchers published a book which showed the original ideas of the California group were now international scientific facts. Although orthodox medical authorities continued to believe theories which were directly contradicted by laboratory demonstrations, the basis for an entirely new approach to cancer research and treatment was a scientifically established reality.

In 1986, an authority in the field summarized the current situation as follows: "Only in the past 2-4 years have microbiologists developed the slightest interest in living microorganisms. When they start truly looking at living microorganisms, the *process* of change taking place before their eyes will confound the problem. We are going to have to teach them what they are seeing. It's a totally different world than what they think they know."

In the past year, a leading scientist from Europe has reexamined the work and the claims of the California group which cured cancer in the 1930s. He concluded, "The principle is sound."

What follows is a complex tale of scientific brilliance and determination by a number of researchers. Sadly, it is also a tale of scientific ignorance, deception, abuse of power, and criminal acts. Congress, the media, and the scientific community should begin public investigations of these matters if the public trust is not to be further eroded.

More than 1,200 Americans will die from cancer in the next 24 hours—nearly one death every minute.

Surely it is time for the suffering to stop.

Chapter 2
Bacteria and Virus

In 19th century France, two giants of science collided. One of them is now world-renowned—Louis Pasteur. The other, from whom Pasteur stole many of his best ideas, is now essentially forgotten—Pierre Bechamp. However, it is possible that as medical knowledge advances and the relationships between health, the immune system, and food patterns are better understood, Bechamp may come to be recognized as the more significant of the two men.

E. Douglas Hume, author of *Bechamp or Pasteur,* asserts that it was Pasteur's faulty science, combined with his public standing, which set the direction of 20th century medicine—chemicals, injections, and experimental transfers of disease cultures from one species to another. According to Hume, medicine could have proceeded in a very different direction if Bechamp's research had received the public attention it deserved. It is now widely recognized that Pasteur was wrong on a number of basic issues.

One of the many areas in which Pasteur and Bechamp argued concerned what is today known as *pleomorphism*—the occurrence of more than one distinct form of an organism in a single life cycle. Bechamp contended that bacteria could change forms. A rod-shaped bacteria could become a spheroid, etc. Pasteur disagreed. In 1914, Madame Victor Henri of the Pasteur Institute confirmed that Bechamp was correct and Pasteur wrong.

But Bechamp went much further in his argument for pleomorphism. He contended that bacteria could "devolve" into smaller, unseen forms, what he called "microzymia." In other words, Bechamp developed—on the basis of a lifetime of research—a theory that micro-organisms could change their essential *size* as well as their shape, depending on the state of health of the organism in which the micro-organism lived. This directly contradicted what orthodox medical authorities have believed for most of the 20th century. Laboratory research in recent years has provided confirmation for Bechamp's notion. An entire century of medicine and scientific research might have been different if Pasteur's public authority and the commercial gains to be realized from his faulty ideas had not predominated.

In 1980, French bacteriologists Sorin Sonea and Maurice Panisset published *A New Bacteriology*. The central theme of their book was that bacterial pleomorphism was now a scientific fact. They stated that "different types of bacteria were only different manifestations of a unified bacteria world."

This seemingly esoteric scientific squabble had ramifications far beyond academic institutions. The denial of pleomorphism was one of the cornerstones of 20th century medical research and cancer treatment. An early 20th century acceptance of pleomorphism might have prevented millions of Americans from suffering and dying of cancer.

In the early third of this century, a heated debate took place over filtrable bacteria versus non-filtrable bacteria. The orthodox view was that bacteria could not be filtered to a smaller form. What passed through "bacteria-proof" filters was something else: not bacteria, but viruses. Standard textbooks today continue to make this same basic distinction between bacteria and viruses.

A "typical" bacteria is about 1 micron in size, or 1/25,000 of an inch. Viruses range in size from 10 millimicrons (10 thousandths of a micron) to 300 millimicrons (300 thousandths of a micron). Thus, the largest virus, according to the orthodox view, is a quarter to a third the size of the average bacteria.

This measurement is important because 300 millimicrons also is the limit of resolution of the light microscope. Viruses require an electron microscope to be seen and electron microscopes kill the specimens. Only the very large smallpox virus can be seen with a light microscope.

Since viruses passed through pores in a filter which held back anything larger than 300 millimicrons, viruses were termed "filtrable viruses" at one time. But eventually the terms "filtrable" and "viruses" became synonymous. A virus was filtrable. But bacteria, according to the orthodox view, could not be filtered to a smaller, earlier stage. Here loomed a major battle in the war over pleomorphism.

Another criterion for a virus is that it requires a living cell as a host in order to reproduce. This fundamental distinction between bacteria and viruses was announced by Dr. Thomas Rivers of the Rockefeller Institute to the Society of American Bacteriologists in December 1926. It helped to establish the foundation for his career as well as to distinguish virology as a separate specialty within the broader field of microbiology. In time, Rivers—because of his scientific reputation, his quarrelsome personality, and the immense financial resources at his disposal through the Rockefeller Institute—became one of the most formidable men in American microbiology. As Director of the Rockefeller Hospital from 1937 to 1955, and as Vice-President of the Rockefeller Institute from 1953 until illness and death removed him from a power role in American medicine, not only did his ideas influence the leading virus researchers of the next generation, but his personal training of a dozen or more of them had a profound impact on research priorities well into the 1970s and 1980s. Unfortunately, Dr. Thomas Rivers was wrong about filtrable bacteria.

A quotation from an article by Dr. Richard Shope which appeared in *The Journal of Bacteriology* in 1962 after the death of Rivers provides some insight into what anyone disagreeing with Rivers would face: "Many of those who have known Dr. Rivers best have felt the sting that he could so picturesquely deliver in an argument. Few of us have had the nerve openly to side with his opposition in one of these 'knock down' and 'drag out' discussions."

But one man who did challenge Rivers was Dr. Arthur Kendall (1877-1959), a noted bacteriologist of his time. Kendall was thoroughly defeated by Rivers as far as public acclaim and orthodox peer recognition was concerned, but just as with

Bechamp in the earlier battle with Pasteur, the science of later generations appears to be reassessing where the true honors should be assigned.

Dr. Arthur Kendall was Director of the Hygienic Laboratory of the Panama Canal Commission in 1904. The Hygienic Laboratory was the forerunner of the National Institute of Health. In 1906, Kendall became a bacteriologist at the Rockefeller Institute. This was followed by 3 years as an instructor at Harvard University Medical School (1909-1912). In 1912, Kendall became head of the first wholly independent Department of Bacteriology in America, at Northwestern University. In 1916, he was appointed Dean of the Medical School. In 1924, Kendall became Professor of Bacteriology and public health at Washington University in St. Louis, Missouri. Then in 1928, he returned to Northwestern and shortly afterwards began working with the California group which conducted the first successful cancer clinic in 1934. In 1942 he retired from Northwestern. More than 100 of his papers were published.

On December 11, 1931, *Science* magazine reported in its Science News section that Dr. Kendall had filtered bacteria to a smaller form and that these micro-organisms had remained alive on a medium of his creation. His "K Medium" had broken down the typhoid bacillus into a filtrable form. Moreover, using a special microscope, he was able to see: (1) the full sized bacillus still unchanged, (2) other bacilli in an intermediate stage between the filtrable and the non-filtrable phases, and (3) still other, very small turquoise-blue bodies which were the final bacillus form. This final form was the size of a virus, and yet it was still a bacteria! The basis for Dr. Rivers' authority had been challenged.

When the official publication of the California Medical Association, *California and Western Medicine,* published the incredible news in December 1931, and Dr. Kendall was invited to address the Association of American Physicians, Rivers reacted. First he tried to have Kendall's talk cancelled. When that was refused by the sponsors, he insisted that he and Dr. Hans Zinsser of Harvard be allowed to speak also. After Kendall made his presentation before the Association in May

1932, Zinsser and Rivers publicly ripped Kendall apart, stating that since they could not replicate Kendall's results, Kendall was lying. The opposition mounted by Rivers and Zinsser was such that few scientists and doctors of the time dared to support Kendall. Kendall could not convince the orthodox "non-filtration" school that experiments done according to his techniques would validate his discovery. The opposition group did not want to learn.

In 1974, Lida H. Mattman of the Department of Biology, Wayne State University, published *Cell-Wall Deficient Forms*. By then, *pleomorphism* was a proven phenomenon although the orthodox school continued to ignore it. Mattman wrote, "Current bacteriology holds the belief that each species of bacteria has only a certain very simple form. . . . In contrast, this writer, using carefully prepared pure cultures, found that bacteria pass through stages with markedly different morphology."

Citing studies that went back more than 30 years, Mattman opened the door to a modern field of research which the existing cancer authorities had not only ignored, but dismissed or suppressed because it conflicted with their own beliefs and their own self-interest.

Mattman, writing with scholarly conservatism, recognized Kendall's contribution and obliquely the erroneous attack on him in the early 1930s: "In the 1920s an important 'school of filtration' was established by Kendall. . . . Although William H. Welch regarded Kendall's work as a distinct advance, great skepticism was expressed on the whole. Unfortunately, this was just prior to the demonstration by Kleineberger and by Dienes that filtrable organisms could be grown on solid medium and their sequential reversion steps followed."

Both Kleineberger and Dienes published their initial findings in the mid-1930s. Kendall was only a few years ahead of them. But Kleineberger and Dienes had no effect either. Something more fundamental was operating, as time would demonstrate. Kendall had not only challenged the experience of Rivers and other established authorities, but had unknowingly threatened medical and financial interests.

By 1982, when Gerald J. Donigue of Tulane University

School of Medicine published *Cell-Wall Deficient Bacteria,* the suppression of Kendall's work for 50 years had obvious results. Domingue writes:

> "There is a considerable body of experimental and clinical evidence—much of which has never been published—supporting the concept that cell wall deficient bacteria may be agents of disease. . . . There are no current books whose primary focus is on the clinical significance of these unusual bodies. . . . The most neglected research area has been on the role of these organisms in disease."

Thus, 50 years after Kendall's discovery, even with substantial evidence, the erroneous orthodox view continued to dominate medical theory, cancer research, and cancer treatment.

One of Kendall's renowned supporters was Dr. Edward Rosenow of the Mayo Clinic. Rosenow was viciously attacked by Thomas Rivers of the rival Rockefeller Institute. As reported in the 1976 article in *New Age Journal,* Rosenow's son, Dr. Edward C. Rosenow, Jr., Chief Administrative Officer of the American College of Physicians, "asserts that his father was all but accused by Rockefeller Institute research moguls of experimental dishonesty."

Rosenow told his son, "They simply won't listen." (Rosenow's son later told how, while a student of Zinsser's at Harvard, Zinsser had admitted to Rosenow Jr. that he, Zinsser, had not even used Rosenow Sr.'s medium in failing to duplicate and then condemning Rosenow's test results.)

The medical moguls apparently wouldn't listen even to one of their own. In 1911, Peyton Rous of the Rockefeller Institute provided the first evidence that a virus could cause a cancer. Yet for decades the orthodox view was that cancer resulted from "somatic mutation"—a gene develops a flaw and disorganizes cellular function.

David Locke, author of a book on viruses published in 1974, recalled meeting Peyton Rous in the corridors of the Rockefeller Institute during the mid-century and being shocked to learn that a micro-organism could be the cause of cancer. Locke wrote, "The 1940s and 1950s were the heyday of the somatic mutation theory. At the time, it was scientific dogma that cancer was a peculiar transformation of cells caused not by an infectious agent, but by a mutation of the cells."

Peyton Rous was finally honored for his discovery in 1966 when he received the Nobel Prize. He was 86 years old and his discovery 55 years past.

Because the Rous virus has been around for so long, it has been carefully categorized. However, as described in Lida Mattman's 1974 book, the Rous "virus" has been found to be a classical bacterium. Citing Dr. Eleanor Alexander-Jackson's work, Mattman explained that the Rous virus produces DNA as well as RNA. Viruses supposedly contain only DNA or RNA, not both.

The orthodox virus school undoubtedly has difficulty with the fact that one of the "classical" viruses—if not the most famous—is in truth a "filtrable bacterium."

In a paper presented to the New York Academy of Sciences in 1969, Dr. Virginia Livingston and Dr. Eleanor Alexander-Jackson declared that a single cancer micro-organism exists. They said that the reason the army of cancer researchers couldn't find it was because it changed form. Livingston and Alexander-Jackson asserted:

"The organism has remained an unclassified mystery, due in part to its remarkable *pleomorphism* and its stimulation of other micro-organisms. Its various phases may resemble viruses, micrococci, diptheroids, bacilli, and fungi."

Florence Seibert, Professor Emeritus of Biochemistry, University of Pennsylvania and Dr. Irene Diller from the Institute for Cancer Research in Philadelphia made essentially the same argument to the New York Academy of Sciences in 1967. Seibert's book *Pebbles on the Hill of a Scientist* (1968) includes the following: "We found that we were able to isolate bacteria from every piece of tumor and every acute leukemic blood specimen that we had. This was published in the Annals of the New York Academy of Sciences."

Seibert also clearly recognized pleomorphism as the underlying scientific reality which must be appreciated if cancer is to be cured:

"One of the most interesting properties of these bacteria is

23

their great pleomorphism. For example, they readily change their shape from round cocci, to elongated rods, and even to long thread-like filaments depending upon what medium they grow on and how long they grow. And even more interesting than this is the fact that these bacteria have a filterable form in their life cycle; that is, that they can become so small that they pass through bacterial filters which hold back bacteria. This is what viruses do, and is one of the main criteria of a virus, separating them from bacteria. But the viruses also will not live on artificial media like these bacteria do. . . . Our filterable form, however, can be recovered again on ordinary artificial bacterial media and will grow on these."

The Mayo Clinic's Dr. Edward Rosenow, who worked with Kendall in the preparatory stage of the successful cancer clinic, had written as early as 1914 in the *Journal of Infectious Diseases* that, "It would seem that focal infections are no longer to be looked upon merely as a place of entrance of bacteria, but as a place where *conditions are favorable for them to acquire the properties* which give them a wide range of affinities for various structures."

This was also Bechamp's conclusion back in the 19th century—that the body's environment produced a place for microorganisms to become diseased bacteria and that improving the body's internal environment could alter bacteria into harmless, even useful "microzymia." E. Douglas Hume has written, "Bechamp . . . had demonstrated the connection between a disturbed state of body and the disturbed state of its indwelling particles, which, upon an unfortunate alteration in their surroundings, are hampered in their normal multiplication as healthy microzymas and are consequently prone to develop into organisms of varied shape, known as bacteria. Upon an improvement in their environment, the bacteria, according to Bechamp's view, by a form of devolution may return to their microzymian state, but much smaller and more numerous than they were originally."

At the end of 1971, Congress passed the National Cancer Act. As Robin and David Nicholas later wrote (*Virology, an Information Profile*) in 1983, "In the 1970s research into the role of viruses in cancer was virtually given a blank check, particularly in the USA, the powerhouse of virus research."

Bacteria and its various forms were ignored. Even in 1986, when researchers mention bacteria as a possible cause of cancer, they are dismissed by the "experts." One high university official stopped reading a report on the 1934 cancer cure when he came across the word bacteria, so brainwashed was he to the certainty that viruses were the cause of cancer while bacteria were of no importance in cancer.

And yet, by 1986, despite the massive fundings of virus research, more people than ever continued to die of cancer. Memorial Sloan-Kettering Cancer Center, the world's largest non-profit cancer research center, and still the leading institutional opponent of pleomorphism research and related cancer treatment in America, stated in a 1986 fund-raising appeal that over 460,000 Americans died of cancer in 1985. (Sloan-Kettering's own 1975 tests had indicated pleomorphic bacteria-virus in *all* cancer blood tests, but they had buried the laboratory results.)

In 1974, Rockefeller University's Dr. Norman Zinder admitted, "We don't know how to attack cancer, much less conquer it, because we don't understand enough about how it works."

Yet the answer existed then and now in scientific journals, Academy of Sciences' reports, books, old newspapers, and other forms. If money wasn't being invested into careful research and cross-referencing of all the relevant literature, then why wasn't it?

The cancer authorities—in the 1980s as in earlier decades—had censored ideas and researchers who argued the unorthodox pleomorphism cause and cure for cancer. The money and clinical trials went to orthodox virus monomorphism supporters and chemical treatments aimed at killing cancerous *cells,* not micro-organisms in the bloodstream attacking the entire body. The funding procedure was essentially stacked against those who, even though top scientists, didn't parrot the conventional (and wrong) beliefs.

Ralph W. Moss, former Assistant Director of Public Affairs at Memorial Sloan-Kettering Cancer Center explained the roadblock in his 1980 book *The Cancer Syndrome:* "A new grant request must therefore be approved by a wide variety of scientists, bureaucrats and businessmen. It must be the result of a *consensus* of opinion among these many individuals. Almost by definition, however, such an application must be well within the bounds of conventional science. These 'cumbersome constraints' make it difficult, if not impossible for radically new ideas to be approved by the NCI." (NCI = the National Cancer Institute)

The "radically new ideas" might include the one that cured cancer in the California clinic in 1934. The 460,000 Americans scheduled to needlessly die in the next year might like some of their tax money to fund a new clinic using those long covered-up ideas and technologies. As Frank J. Rauscher, Jr., Director of the National Cancer Institute, rhetorically asked in 1975, "What are we doing with the taxpayer's money?"

It is a question which no one in authority wants to answer honestly—the horrible results of the cancer cure cover-up are too well-known. The death toll from 1970 to the present (1986) is more than 6 million, matching the Nazi holocaust. When the death count includes those who died from 1934 to 1970, the number of victims is staggering. The cancer cure cover-up is America's holocaust.

A political firestorm could erupt if a large sector of the American public learned the truth.

Chapter 3

Medicine in America

The suppression of the successful cancer cure first used in 1934 took place because of a unique set of factors. Among these factors were: the virtual one-man rule within the American Medical Association, scientific rivalries, institutional pride and arrogance, a power-hungry head at Memorial Sloan-Kettering determined to find his own cure for cancer even if it required squashing those with different views, pharmaceutical companies with vested interests which slowly took control of the direction of America's cancer program, and political-media timidity in the area of medical oversight. There were a number of junctures during the years since 1934 when, if one person in a critical position had acted courageously, the entire history of medicine in this century could have been altered. But it didn't happen. The resulting cost in lives and resources has been incalculable. It is not an exaggeration to say that the cover-up, suppression, and failure to evaluate the 1934 cancer cure has been an American catastrophe exceeding anything in our history. Even if the 1934 cure can be implemented in the late 1980s, nothing can disguise the waste and horror of what has happened.

The American Medical Association was formed in 1846, but it wasn't until 1901 that a reorganization enabled it to gain power over how medicine was practiced throughout America. By becoming a confederation of state medical associations and forcing doctors who wanted to belong to their county medical society to join the state association, the AMA soon increased its membership to include a majority of physicians. Then, by accrediting medical schools, it began determining the standards and practices of doctors. Those who refused to conform lost their license to practice medicine.

In 1912 the AMA established its "cooperative" advertising bureau. Soon the AMA's Chicago headquarters determined not only who could advertise in the state medical journals but how much advertisers were expected to pay if their products were to be "approved." Morris Fishbein was the virtual dictator of the AMA from the mid-1920s until he was ousted on June 6, 1949 at the AMA convention in Atlantic City. But even after he was forced from his position of power because of a revolt from several state delegations of doctors, the policies he had set in motion continued on for many years. He died in the early 1970s.

The Illinois Medical Society had warned as early as 1922 about what was happening, but few paid attention or dared to oppose the trend: "The AMA is a one-man organization. The entire medical profession of the United States is at the mercy of one man. . . . The Journal controls all the funds."

One example demonstrates how the AMA advertising and approval "racket" worked. According to Morris A. Beale, author of two books, *The Super Drug Story* and *Medical Mussolini,* C. Gildner of Los Angeles contracted with King's Laboratories to distribute a product called Maelum. King's Laboratories requested approval by the AMA for its product. On October 27, 1931, AMA director Fishbein wrote that it was approved. On November 10, 1931, Gildner was approached by Fishbein to purchase advertising in the national AMA Journal or any of the 42 state medical journals. Gildner refused. On November 16, 1931, one week later, through the AMA's Committee on Foods, Fishbein revoked the AMA's seal of approval.

According to Beale, this procedure was common practice. Products weren't tested for their effects on health. Only advertising revenues were considered. In short, the AMA for many years was abusing its position of power to shake down potential advertisers. Even worse, it was selling its product approval seal to advertisers whose products were unsafe and unhealthy. Products virtually the same would be found on the AMA's "approved" and "disapproved" lists—the only distinction being whether their manufacturers advertised in the Journal of the AMA.

The man responsible for this state of affairs was, in the words of Associated Press Science Writer Howard Blakeslee, "Morris Fishbein, the Kingpin of American Medicine." Fishbein operated out of the AMA's Chicago headquarters.

A few years after the successful cancer clinic of 1934, Dr. R. T. Hamer, who did not participate in the clinic, began to use the procedure in Southern California. According to Benjamin Cullen, who observed the entire development of the cancer cure from idea to implementation, Fishbein found out and tried to "buy in." When he was turned down, Fishbein unleashed the AMA to destroy the cancer cure.

Cullen recalled: "Dr. Hamer ran an average of forty cases a day through his place. He had to hire two operators. He trained them and watched them very closely. The case histories were mounting up very fast. Among them was this old man from Chicago. He had a malignancy all around his face and neck. It was a gory mass. Just terrible. Just a red gory mass. It had taken over all around his face. It had taken off one eyelid at the bottom of the eye. It had taken off the bottom of the lower lobe of the ear and had also gone into the cheek area, nose and chin. He was a sight to behold."

"But in six months all that was left was a little black spot on the side of his face and the condition of that was such that it was about to fall off. Now that man was 82 years of age. I never saw anything like it. The delight of having a lovely clean skin again, just like a baby's skin."

"Well he went back to Chicago. Naturally he couldn't keep still and Fishbein heard about it. Fishbein called him in and the old man was kind of reticent about telling him. So Fishbein wined and dined him and finally learned about his cancer treatment by Dr. Hamer in the San Diego clinic."

"Well soon a man from Los Angeles came down. He had several meetings with us. Finally he took us out to dinner and broached the subject about buying it. Well we wouldn't do it. The renown was spreading and we weren't even advertising. But of course what did it was the case histories of Dr. Hamer. He said that this was the most marvelous development of the age. His case histories were absolutely wonderful."

"Fishbein bribed a partner in the company. With the result

we were kicked into court—operating without a license. I was broke after a year."

In 1939, under pressure from the local medical society, Dr. R. T. Hamer abandoned the cure. He is not one of the heroes of this story.

Thus, within the few, short years from 1934 to 1939, the cure for cancer was clinically demonstrated and expanded into curing other diseases on a daily basis by other doctors, and then terminated when Morris Fishbein of the AMA was not allowed to "buy in." It was a practice he had developed into a cold art, but never again would such a single mercenary deed doom millions of Americans to premature, ugly deaths. It was the AMA's most shameful hour. In years to come, it may be the event which triggers lawsuits against the AMA for damages exceeding anything in American legal history.

Where was the federal government at this time (1938-1939)? Just getting organized. The Hygienic Laboratory was reorganized into the National Institutes of Health in 1930, but in 1938 it was in the process of moving into its permanent location outside Washington, D.C. in Bethesda, Maryland. The National Institutes of Health were a small operation then. The National Cancer Institute had been created only in 1937. Government grants to cure cancer were only beginning. And in 1938, Fishbein was in Washington, D.C. lobbying to stop Roosevelt's first effort to establish a national health program. Keeping the government out of the health business as well as keeping outsiders with a lasting cure for cancer "out in the cold" were the objectives of those who then had a monopoly on medicine.

The insiders included two other groups—the private research centers and the pharmaceutical companies. Paul Starr explained the situation in his 1984 Pulitzer Prize book, *The Social Transformation of Medicine:*

"Between 1900 and 1940, the primary sources of financing for medical research were private. Private foundations and universities were the principal sponsors and hosts of basic research. The most richly endowed research center, the Rockefeller Institute for Medical Research, was established in 1902 and by 1928 had received from John D. Rockefeller $65 million in endowment funds."

30

"The other major private sponsors of research were pharmaceutical companies, which grew rapidly after the 1920s. . . . An estimate in 1945 put the research expenditures of the drug companies at $40 million, compared to $25 million for the foundations, universities, and research institutes."

Another major institution which "staked its claim" in the virgin territory of cancer research in the 1930-1950 period was Memorial Sloan-Kettering Cancer Center in New York. Established in 1884 as the first cancer hospital in America, Memorial Sloan-Kettering from 1940 to the mid-1950s was the center of drug testing for the largest pharmaceutical companies. Cornelius P. Rhoads, who had spent the 1930s at the Rockefeller Institute, became the director at Memorial Sloan-Kettering in 1939. He remained in that position until his death in 1959. Rhoads was the head of the chemical warfare service from 1943-1945, and afterwards became the nation's premier advocate of chemotherapy. According to Dr. Virginia Livingston-Wheeler, "Dr. Rhoads was determined to dictate the cancer policies of the entire country."

It was Dr. Rhoads who prevented Dr. Irene Diller from announcing the discovery of the cancer micro-organism to the New York Academy of Sciences in 1950. It also was Dr. Rhoads who arranged for the funds for Dr. Caspe's New Jersey laboratory to be cancelled after she announced the same discovery in Rome in 1953. And an I.R.S. investigation, instigated by an unidentified, powerful New York cancer authority, added to her misery. The laboratory was closed.

Memorial Sloan-Kettering is closely tied to the American Cancer Society. The American Cancer Society was founded in 1913 by John D. Rockefeller, Jr. and his business associates. Reorganized after the war, the power positions on its board were taken by pharmaceutical executives, advertising people, Sloan-Kettering trustees, and other orthodox treatment proponents. The American Cancer Society has enormous influence in the cancer world because its public appeals generate large amounts of money for research. As Ralph W. Moss, former Assistant Director of Public Affairs at Memorial Sloan-Kettering Cancer Center, made explicit, "The Society now has tens of millions of dollars to distribute to those who favor its growing power, and many powerful connections to disconcert those who oppose it."

Yet with all this wealth at its disposal for so many years, and its purpose the eradication of cancer, the American Cancer Society has not been able to find those scientists who have scientifically isolated the cancer micro-organism or those pioneer researchers and doctors who cured it in 1934 and afterwards. Bad luck, incompetence, or something else?

Thus the major players on the cancer field are the doctors, the private research institutions, the pharmaceutical companies, the American Cancer Society, and also the U.S. government through the National Cancer Institute (organizing research) and the Food and Drug Administration (the dreaded FDA which keeps the outsiders on the defensive through raids, legal harassment, and expensive testing procedures).

The people in these institutions, and especially their political management, all proclaim their professionalism, dedication, and expertise. The results tell a very different story. Ralph Moss exposes the chink in the cancer establishment's armor with a single quotation in *The Cancer Syndrome*. It is by the late Sloan-Kettering chemotherapist David Karnofsky: "The relevant matter in examining any form of treatment is not the reputation of its proponent, the persuasiveness of his theory, the eminence of its lay supporters, the testimony of patients, or the existence of public controversy, but simply— does the treatment work?"

If only Rivers, Fishbein, Rhoads and the army of current skeptical research-oriented scientists, bureaucrats, pharmaceutical spokesmen, philanthropists and other credentialed professionals had honored the scientific and moral rightness of Karnofsky's thought, the cure for cancer might not have been suppressed for decades and might have a chance for a swift testing and implementation today.

David M. Locke emphasized the same point as Karnofsky in the book *Viruses:*

> "One of the dicta of the University of Chicago's great cancer researcher and Nobel Laureate, Charles B. Huggins, is: 'The thing about cancer is to cure it.'"

32

Chapter 4

The Man Who Found
The Cure For Cancer

In 1913, a man with a love for machines and a scientific curiosity arrived in San Diego after driving across the country from New York. He had been born in Elkhorn, Nebraska, was 25 years old, and very happily married. He was about to start a new life and open the way to a science of health which will be honored far into the future. His name was Royal Raymond Rife. Close friends, who loved his gentleness and humility while being awed by his genius, called him Roy.

Royal R. Rife was fascinated by bacteriology, microscopes and electronics. For the next 7 years (including a mysterious period in the Navy during World War I in which he traveled to Europe to investigate foreign laboratories for the U.S. government), he thought about and experimented in a variety of fields as well as mastered the mechanical skills necessary to build instruments such as the world had never imagined.

So it was that, in 1920 when the great idea of his life came to him, Royal Rife was ready. Journalist Newall Jones described the historic moment in the May 6, 1938 *Evening Tribune* of San Diego:

"The San Diego man, who is hailed by many as a veritable genius, has experimented with important studies, inventions and discoveries in an unbelievably wide and varied array of subjects. These fields of pursuit range from ballistics and racing auto construction to optics and many equally profound sciences. And in 1920 he was investigating the possibilities of electrical treatment of diseases.

"It was then that he noticed these individualistic differences in the chemical constituents of disease organisms and saw the indication of electrical characteristics, observed electrical polarities in the organisms.

33

> "Random speculation on the observation suddenly stirred in his mind a startling, astonishing thought.
>
> "'What would happen if I subjected these organisms to different electrical frequencies?' he wondered."

So he began to gather the tools necessary to do so: microscopes, electronic equipment, tubes, bacteriological equipment, cages for guinea pigs, cameras, and machinery to build his own designs. Two San Diego industrialists—Timken, owner of the Timken Roller Bearing Company and Bridges, owner of the Bridges Carriage Company—provided funds to establish a laboratory and finance Rife's research.

By the late 1920s, the first phase of his work was completed. He had built his first microscope, one that broke the existing principles, and he had constructed instruments which enabled him to electronically destroy specific pathological micro-organisms.

In the years that followed, he would improve and perfect these early models, identify and classify disease-causing micro-organisms in a totally unique way, including their exact M.O.R. or Mortal Oscillatory Rate (the precise frequency which "blew them up") and then, in cooperation with leading bacteriologists such as Rosenow and Kendall, along with leading doctors, cure cancer and other diseases in people.

Every step was controversial, original, difficult and time-consuming. The opposition was powerful. They eventually did break him and many of those who collaborated with him, but not before Rife left records, microscopes, electronic frequency instruments, and methods which will enable later generations to establish an entirely new form of painless, non-drug healing.

As one of Rife's co-workers recalled in 1958, forty-five years after he met the genius of San Diego:

> "He finally got to a point where from years of isolation and clarification and purification of these filterable forms, he could produce cancer in the guinea pigs in two weeks. He tried it on rats, guinea pigs and rabbits, but he found finally that he could confine his efforts to guinea pigs and white rats because every doggone one was his pet. And he performed the operations on them in the most meticulous operations you ever want to see in all your born days. No doctor could ever come near to it.

He had to wear a big powerful magnifying glass. He performed the most wonderful operations you ever saw. Completely eradicating every tentacle out from the intestines, and sewed the thing up and it got well and didn't know anything about it at all. Did it not once but hundreds of times. This is a thing that again and again I wish was published. I wish with all my heart that all the detailed information that he developed could be published because the man deserves it.

"He finally got these cultures on the slide. He could look through this thing and you could see them swimming around absolutely motile and active. Then he'd say, 'Watch that.' He'd go turn on the frequency lamps. When it got to a certain frequency, he'd release the whole doggone flood of power into the room. The doggone little things would die instantly.

"He built the microscopes himself. He built the micro-manipulator himself. And the micro-dissector and a lot of other stuff.

"I've seen Roy sit in that doggone seat without moving, watching the changes in the frequency, watching when the time would come when the virus in the slide would be destroyed. Twenty-four hours was nothing for him. Forty-eight hours. He had done it many times. Sit there without moving. He wouldn't touch anything except a little water. His nerves were just like cold steel. He never moved. His hands never quivered.

"Of course he would train beforehand and go through a very careful workout afterward to build himself up again. But that is what I would call one of the most magnificent sights of human control and endurance I'd ever seen.

"I've seen the cancer virus. I have seen the polio virus. I've seen the TB virus. Here was a man showing people, showing doctors, these viruses of many different kinds of diseases, especially those three deadly ones—TB, polio and cancer.

"Time and time again since that time some of these medical men have made the proud discovery that they had isolated we will say one of the viruses of cancer, had isolated one of the viruses of polio. Why that was one of the most ridiculous things in the world. Thirty-five years ago Roy Rife showed them these things.

"These machines demonstrate that you could cure cancer— all crazy notions of usurping the rights of the AMA notwithstanding. They definitely could take a leaf out of Roy Rife's book and do an awful lot of good to this world for

35

sickness and disease. As a consequence, we have lost millions of people that could have been healed by Rife's machines.

"I like Roy Rife. I'll always remember Roy as my Ideal. He has a tremendous capacity for knowledge and a tremendous capacity for remembering what he has learned. He definitely was my Ideal. Outside of old Teddy Roosevelt, I don't know of any man any smarter than him and I'll bank him up against a hundred doctors because he did know his stuff with his scientific knowledge in so many lines. He had so many wrinkles that he could have cashed in and made millions out of it if he had wanted to and I do mean millions of dollars. Which would have benefited the human race, irrespective of this tremendous thing that he built which we call the Rife ray machine.

"In my estimation Roy was one of the most gentle, genteel, self-effacing, moral men I ever met. Not once in all the years I was going over there to the lab, and that was approximately 30 years, did I ever hear him say one word out of place.

"All the doctors used to beat a path to Rife's lab door and that was a beautiful lab at one time. It was beautifully arranged inside. The equipment was just exactly right; his study was just wonderful. It was a place of relics and the atmosphere could not be duplicated anywhere."

Chapter 5
The 1920s

Rife began in 1920 by searching for an electronic means to destroy the micro-organism which caused tuberculosis. It was in that first year that the original radio frequency instrument was built. Since the frequency which would kill the micro-organism was unknown, Rife had to proceed by trial and error. Rife and his associates conducted test after test.

Finally he achieved success, but the success produced more problems. The micro-organism had been killed, but in several cases the guinea pigs died of toxic poisoning. Three years were spent in finding an answer. He suspected that a virus from the bacteria was responsible. He would have to devise a way to obtain the virus in pure form in order to determine its frequency and thus kill it without injuring the pigs.

Rife's first microscope also was completed in 1920 although he began building it in 1917. From 1920 to 1925, some 20,000 pathological tissues were sectioned and stained. However, they failed to show any unknown bacteria or foreign material under the highest power. Rife continued to improve it, searching for a way to see the viruses.

He knew about the 19th century work of Voghn and later Robert Cook who were able to destroy the rod form of the tuberculosis bacteria with vaccine and anti-toxins, but still were left with experimental animals which died. Rife theorized that they had released the virus by killing the bacteria—just as he had done when he destroyed the Bacillus of Tuberculosis with his radio frequency instrument. Unless he could see the virus and determine its frequency, he couldn't cure TB with his method. But if he could see in his microscope both the bacterial and the viral forms of TB, he could determine their separate frequencies and kill them both at the same time.

Rife believed that the minuteness of the viruses made it impossible to stain them with the existing acid or aniline dye stains. He'd have to find another way. Somewhere along the way, he made an intuitive leap often associated with the greatest scientific discoveries. He conceived first the idea and then the method of staining the virus with *light*. He began building a microscope which would enable a frequency of light to coordinate with the chemical constituents of the particle or microorganism under observation.

Rife later explained to a reporter how he was able to make this leap. In a front page article of the San Diego Union on November 3, 1929, Rife is quoted, "If one man is a bacteriologist and knows what is needed and another is a mechanic who tries to build it, they may get somewhere, but they will do it slowly and imperfectly. But if both these men are the same man he will know the set-up from both angles; then if you add delicacy, accuracy, mechanical skill, the willingness to keep proper records, ingenuity and the patience to learn from failures, you will be well along toward the solution of your problem and the perfection of the necessary apparatus, whatever it is."

Rife's second microscope was finished in 1929. In an article which appeared in the *Los Angeles Times Magazine* on December 27, 1931, the existence of the light staining method was reported to the public:

> "Bacilli may thus be studied by their light, exactly as astronomers study moons, suns, and stars by the light which comes from them through telescopes. The bacilli studied are living ones, not corpses killed by stains."

Throughout most of this period, Rife also had been seeking a way to identify and then destroy the micro-organism which caused cancer. His cancer research began in 1922. It would take him until 1932 to isolate the responsible micro-organism which he later named simply the "BX virus."

The 1920s were the years of pure isolated research for Rife. There were no famous microbiologists coming to his door, no doctors seeking to use his frequency instrument on their patients, no requests from microscope experts to be allowed to learn about his invention, no medical committees established to coordinate the laboratory and clinical results, no renowned cancer experts negotiating to work with him in his lab, no cancer foundations trying to fit his discoveries into their grant procedures. But all the scientific isolation was to end soon after the microscope's existence was reported in 1929.

Rife would have to make time for experimental demonstrations, letters, and meetings. He'd have to deal with more people, and still preserve time for the exhausting research which only he could do because only he knew how to do it. Others could help, and they did, but they also got in the way. Then there would be the businessmen promoters and doctors who would try to steal his work. There would be the opposition from scientists whose own authority, prestige, and position would be challenged by Rife's discoveries. And there would be the powerful attempt by Morris Fishbein and the AMA to destroy the man whose miraculous treatment they could not "buy into".

So in retrospect the 1920s seem to be some of Rife's most frustrating years as he struggled to find answers. But in another sense, they were his golden years of what he called "pure science".

On November 3, 1929, the *San Diego Union* carried a front page article titled "Local Man Bares Wonders of Germ Life." The article described the wonders Rife could accomplish with his new microscope. It announced that Rife's "light staining" method was nearing perfection. The article explained:

"He holds a theory that the harsh acid stains used to bring out features of the tissue, as well as the complicated treatment now necessary to prepare it for the slides, conspire to defeat their own objective.

"He believes that the chemical baths themselves destroy the very germ that science is trying to pin under the microscope.

"So he is evolving a new method that will do away with chemicals. Instead of five days' hard work being necessary before a pickled and probably worthless section of tissue can be put under the lens, he expects within three minutes to place a perfectly normal, undoped slice of the diseased substance in position for examination.

"The possibilities of this process once it is perfected, he

believes are boundless. Medical men who for all time have been destroying the very thing they were looking for, while they were getting ready to look at it, may in this one step find an end to much of human suffering."

The roaring 20s were over. Two weeks before the first newspaper article, the stock market had crashed. A decade of depression lay ahead for America. And Rife's fabulous discoveries, inventions, and health miracles would have to contend not only with professional scientific skepticism and a powerful medical union determined to control the health business, but also with the national economic crisis which made financing research a difficult and complicated challenge.

Yet his primary goal would be accomplished. The cancer micro-organism would be isolated and destroyed. Terminally ill cancer patients would be treated. And they would be healed. Rife would do what he had set out to do. It would be decades before his work would be recognized. But the "pure science" he accomplished meant the deadly BX cancer micro-organism someday would be "blown up" in those suffering from its effects.

Chapter 6

The Early 1930s

In 1931, the two men who provided the greatest professional support to Royal R. Rife came into his life. Dr. Arthur I. Kendall was Director of Medical Research at Northwestern University Medical School in Illinois. Dr. Milbank Johnson was a member of the board of directors at Pasadena Hospital in California and an influential power in Los Angeles medical circles. Together, Rife, Kendall and Johnson slowly and carefully began an assault on the scientific and medical orthodoxies of their time.

Probably because of the November 3, 1929 news article in the San Diego Union, Dr. Kendall had learned about Rife's wonder microscope. He asked his friend Dr. Johnson of Los Angeles if such a microscope truly existed. Dr. Johnson and Dr. Alvin G. Foord, the pathologist at Pasadena Hospital (and later President of the American Association of Pathologists), journeyed to San Diego along with two other doctors. Foord's presence from the beginning is important because later he lied about his participation in the great scientific endeavor which followed. By the 1950s the AMA and the California State Board of Public Health were committed to squelching the Rife cancer cure. By then many millions of people had died because the cancer cure had been suppressed, doctors who had used the instrument successfully were being persecuted, and those with reputations to preserve were literally "lying through their teeth" as documents and personal testimony show.

But in 1931 when Johnson and Foord first met Rife, the future seemed to hold only endless medical advances because of Rife's wonderful microscope. The four doctors were impressed. Johnson returned to Los Angeles and wired a report to Kendall in Chicago. Kendall sent a telegram back, "Expect to start for California Saturday night."

Dr. Kendall had invented a protein culture medium (called "K Medium" after its inventor) which enabled the "filtrable virus" portions of a bacteria to be isolated and to continue reproducing. This claim directly contradicted the Rockefeller Institute's Dr. Thomas Rivers who in 1926 had authoritatively stated that a virus needed a living tissue for reproduction. Rife, Kendall and others were to prove within a year that it was possible to cultivate viruses artificially. Rivers, in his ignorance and obstinacy, was responsible for suppressing one of the greatest advances ever made in medical knowledge.

Of course, when Rivers opposed Kendall in 1932 and called him a liar at the meeting of the Association of American Physicians in Baltimore, Rivers had not had the opportunity to see the viruses on the "K Medium" under Rife's microscope. But Rivers wasn't interested in learning about the microscope, even after other top bacteriologists saw the same results. Rivers' mistaken notion is still "law" in orthodox circles of the 1980s.

Kendall arrived in California in mid-November 1931 and Johnson introduced him to Rife. Kendall brought his "K Medium" to Rife and Rife brought his microscope to Kendall. A meeting of historic importance took place.

A typhoid germ was put in the "K Medium," triple-filtered through the finest filter available, and the results examined under Rife's microscope. Tiny, distinct bodies stained in a turquoise-blue light were visible. Kendall could "see" the proof of what he had demonstrated by other means. Two historic breakthroughs in science had happened. The virus cultures grew in the "K Medium" and were visible. The viruses could be "light" stained and then classified according to their own colors under Rife's unique microscope.

A later report which appeared in the Smithsonian's annual publication gives a hint of the totally original microscopic technology which enabled man to see a deadly virus-size micro-organism in its live state for the first time (the electron microscope of later years kills its specimens):

"Then they were examined under the Rife microscope where

the filterable virus form of typhoid bacillus, emitting a blue spectrum color, caused the plane of polarization to be deviated 4.8 degrees plus. When the opposite angle of refraction was obtained by means of adjusting the polarizing prisms to minus 4.8 degrees and the cultures of viruses were illuminated by the monochromatic beams coordinated with the chemical constituents of the typhoid bacillus, small, oval, actively motile, bright turquoise-blue bodies were observed at $5000 \times$ magnification, in high contrast to the colorless and motionless debris of the medium. These tests were repeated 18 times to verify the results."

Following the success, Dr. Milbank Johnson quickly arranged a dinner in honor of the two men in order that the discovery could be announced and discussed. More than 30 of the most prominent medical doctors, pathologists, and bacteriologists in Los Angeles attended this historic event on November 20, 1931. Among those in attendance were Dr. Alvin G. Foord who 20 years later would indicate he knew little about Rife's discoveries and Dr. George Dock who would serve on the University of Southern California's Special Research Committee overseeing the clinical work until he, too, would "go over" to the opposition.

On November 22, 1931, the *Los Angeles Times* reported this important medical gathering and its scientific significance:

"Scientific discoveries of the greatest magnitude, including a discussion of the world's most powerful microscope recently perfected after 14 years effort by Dr. Royal R. Rife of San Diego, were described Friday evening to members of the medical profession, bacteriologists and pathologists at a dinner given by Dr. Milbank Johnson in honor of Dr. Rife and Dr. A. I. Kendall.

"Before the gathering of distinguished men, Dr. Kendall told of his researches in cultivating the typhoid bacillus on his new 'K Medium.' The typhoid bacillus is nonfilterable and is large enough to be seen easily with microscopes in general use. Through the use of 'medium K,' Dr. Kendall said, the organism is so altered that it cannot be seen with ordinary microscopes and it becomes small enough to be ultra-microscopic or filterable. It then can be changed back to the microscopic or non-filterable form.

"Through the use of Dr. Rife's powerful microscope, said

43

to have a visual power of magnification to 17,000 times, compared with 2000 times of which the ordinary microscope is capable, Dr. Kendall said he could see the typhoid bacilli in the filterable or formerly invisible stage. It is probably the first time the minute filterable (virus) organisms ever have been seen.

"The strongest microscope now in use can magnify between 2000 and 2500 times. Dr. Rife, by an ingenious arrangement of lenses applying an entirely new optical principle and by introducing double quartz prisms and powerful illuminating lights, has devised a microscope with a lowest magnification of 5,000 times and a maximum working magnification of 17,000 times.

"The new microscope, scientists predict, also will prove a development of the first magnitude. Frankly dubious about the perfection of a microscope which appears to transcend the limits set by optic science, Dr. Johnson's guests expressed themselves as delighted with the visual demonstration and heartily accorded both Dr. Rife and Dr. Kendall a foremost place in the world's rank of scientists."

Five days later, the *Los Angeles Times* published a photo of Rife and Kendall with the microscope. It was the first time a picture of the super microscope had appeared in public. The headline read, "The World's Most Powerful Microscope."

Meanwhile, Rife and Kendall had prepared an article for the December 1931 issue of *California and Western Medicine*. "Observations on Bacillus Typhosus in its Filtrable State" described what Rife and Kendall had done and seen. The journal was the official publication of the state medical associations of California, Nevada and Utah.

The prestigious *Science* magazine then carried an article which alerted the scientific community of the entire nation. The December 11, 1931 *Science News* supplement included a section titled, "Filtrable Bodies Seen With The Rife Microscope." The article described Kendall's filtrable medium culture, the turquoise blue bodies which were the filtered form of the typhoid bacillus, and Rife's microscope. It included the following description:

"The light used with Dr. Rife's microscope is polarized, that is, it is passing through crystals that stop all rays except those vibrating in one particular plane. By means of a double reflecting prism built into the instrument, it is possible to turn this plane of vibration in any desired direction, controlling the illumination of the minute objects in the field very exactly."

On December 27, 1931, the *Los Angeles Times* reported that Rife had demonstrated the microscope at a meeting of 250 scientists. The article explained, "This is a new kind of magnifier, and the laws governing microscopes may not apply to it. . . . Dr. Rife has developed an instrument that may revolutionize laboratory methods and enable bacteriologists, like Dr. Kendall, to identify the germs that produce about 50 diseases whose causes are unknown . . . then to find ways and means of immunizing mankind against them."

Soon Kendall was invited to speak before the Association of American Physicians. The presentation occurred May 3 and 4, 1932 at Johns Hopkins University in Baltimore. And there Dr. Thomas Rivers and Hans Zinsser stopped the scientific process. Their opposition meant that the development of Rife's discoveries would be slowed. Professional microbiologists would be cautious in even conceding the possibility that Rife and Kendall might have broken new ground. The depression was at its worst. The Rockefeller Institute was not only a source of funding but powerful in the corridors of professional recognition. A great crime resulted because of the uninformed, cruel and unscientific actions of Rivers and Zinsser.

The momentum was slowed at the moment when Rife's discoveries could have "broken out" and triggered a chain reaction of research, clinical treatment and the beginnings of an entirely new health system. By the end of 1932, Rife could destroy the typhus bacteria, the polio virus, the herpes virus, the cancer virus and other viruses in a culture and in experimental animals. Human treatment was only a step away.

The opposition of Rivers and Zinsser in 1932 had a devastating impact on the history of 20th century medicine. (Zinsser's *Bacteriology* in an updated version is still a standard textbook.) Unfortunately, there were few esteemed bacteriologists who were not frightened or awed by Rivers.

But there were two exceptions to this generally unheroic crowd. Christopher Bird's article "What Has Become Of The

45

Rife Microscope?" which appeared in the March 1976 *New Age Journal,* reports:

> "In the midst of the venom and acerbity the only colleague to come to Kendall's aid was the grand old man of bacteriology, and first teacher of the subject in the United States, Dr. William H. 'Popsy' Welch, who evidently looked upon Kendall's work with some regard."

Welch was the foremost pathologist in America at one time. The medical library at Johns Hopkins University is named after him. He rose and said, "Kendall's observation marks a distinct advance in medicine." It did little good. By then Rivers and Zinsser were the powers in the field.

Kendall's other supporter was Dr. Edward C. Rosenow of the Mayo Clinic's Division of Experimental Bacteriology. (The Mayo Clinic was then and is today one of the outstanding research and treatment clinics in the world. The Washington Post of January 6, 1987 wrote, "To many in the medical community, the Mayo Clinic is 'the standard' against which other medical centers are judged.") On July 5-7, 1932, just two months after Kendall's public humiliation, the Mayo Clinic's Rosenow met with Kendall and Rife at Kendall's Laboratory at Northwestern University Medical School in Chicago.

"The oval, motile, turquoise-blue virus were demonstrated and shown unmistakably," Rosenow declared in the "Proceedings of the Staff Meetings of the Mayo Clinic, July 13, 1932, Rochester, Minnesota." The virus for herpes was also seen. On August 26, 1932, *Science* magazine published Rosenow's report, "Observations with the Rife Microscope of Filter Passing Forms of Micro-organisms."

In the article, Rosenow stated:

> "There can be no question of the filtrable turquoise blue bodies described by Kendall. They are not visible by the ordinary methods of illumination and magnification. . . . Examination under the Rife microscope of specimens, containing objects visible with the ordinary microscope, leaves no doubt of the accurate visualization of objects or particulate matter by direct observation at the extremely high magnification (calculated to be 8,000 diameters) obtained with this instrument."

Three days after departing from Rife in Chicago, Rosenow wrote to Rife from the Mayo Clinic:

"After seeing what your wonderful microscope will do, and after pondering over the significance of what you revealed with its use during those three strenuous and memorable days spent in Dr. Kendall's laboratory, I hope you will take the necessary time to describe how you obtain what physicists consider the impossible. . . . As I visualize the matter, your ingenious method of illumination with the intense monochromatic beam of light is of even greater importance than the enormously high magnification. . . ."

Rosenow was right. The unique "color frequency" staining method was the great breakthrough. Years later, after the arrival of television, an associate of the then deceased Rife would explain, "The viruses were stained with the frequency of light just like colors are tuned in on television sets." It was the best non-technical description ever conceived.

But in 1932, Rife was not interested in writing a scientific paper explaining the physics of his microscope, as Rosenow had hoped. Rife's meeting with Kendall had provided Rife with the "K Medium." And Rife knew what he wanted to do with it. He wanted to find the cancer virus. And that is exactly what he did in 1932.

Chapter 7
"BX"—The Virus of Cancer

Rife began using Kendall's "K Medium" in 1931 in his search for the cancer virus. In 1932, he obtained an unulcerated breast mass that was checked for malignancy from the Paradise Valley Sanitarium of National City, California. But the initial cancer cultures failed to produce the virus he was seeking.

Then a fortuitous accident occurred. The May 11, 1938 *Evening Tribune* of San Diego later described what happened:

"But neither the medium nor the microscope were sufficient alone to reveal the filter-passing organism Rife found in cancers, he recounted. It was an added treatment which he found virtually by chance that finally made this possible, he related. He happened to test a tube of cancer culture within the circle of a tubular ring filled with argon gas activated by an electrical current, which he had been using in experimenting with electronic bombardment of organisms of disease. His cancer culture happened to rest there about 24 hours (with the current on the argon gas filled tube), and then he noticed (under the microscope) that its appearance seemed to have changed. He studied and tested this phenomenon repeatedly, and thus discovered (cancer virus) filter-passing, red-purple granules in the cultures."

Later he perfected this procedure—cancer culture in "K Medium" followed by the argon treatment with the gas-filled tube lighted for 24 hours by a 5000 volt electric current. Then it was placed in a water bath with 2 inches of vacuum and incubated for 24 hours at 37.5 degrees Centigrade. Rife believed the gas-filled tube ionized the cancer culture and this was counteracted by the oxidation in the water vacuum. Some chemical constituents of the organism were so changed that it was brought within the visible spectrum, as seen through Rife's microscope.

The BX cancer virus was a distinct purplish red color. Rife had succeeded in isolating the filtrable virus of carcinoma.

Rife's laboratory notes for November 20, 1932 contain the first written description of the cancer virus characteristics. Among them are two unique to his method of classification using the Rife microscope:

angle of refraction   12-3/10 degrees
color by chemical refraction   purple-red

When Rife copyrighted his discovery in 1953, the angle had changed to 12-3/16 degrees. Perhaps that was his intent all along and the notes were hastily written.

The size of the cancer virus was indeed small. The length was 1/15 of a micron. The breadth was 1/20 of a micron. No ordinary light microscope, even in the 1980s, would be able to make the cancer virus visible.

Rife and his laboratory assistant E. S. Free proceeded to confirm his discovery. They repeated the method 104 consecutive times with identical results.

In time, Rife was able to prove that the cancer micro-organism had 4 forms:

1) BX (carcinoma)
2) BY (sarcoma—larger than BX)
3) Monococcoid form in the monocytes of the blood of over 90% of cancer patients. When properly stained, this form can be readily seen with a standard research microscope
4) Crytomyces pleomorphia fungi—identical morphologically to that of the orchid and of the mushroom

Rife wrote in his 1953 book: "Any of these forms can be changed back to 'BX' within a period of 36 hours and will produce in the experimental animal a typical tumor with all the pathology of true neoplastic tissue, from which we can again recover the 'BX' micro-organism. This complete process has been duplicated over 300 times with identical and positive results."

Rife continued: "After one year, we take this same stock culture of dormant crytomyces pleomorphis fungi and plant it back on its own asparagus base media; there is no longer a crytomyces pleomorphia, no longer a monococcoid organism such as is found in the monocytes of blood, there is no longer a 'BX' or 'BY' form, but there is, from the initial virus isolated directly from an unulcerated human breast mass, a *bacillus coli,* that will pass any known laboratory methods of analysis."

Rife had proved *pleomorphism*. He had shown how the cancer virus changes form, depending on its environment. He had confirmed the work of Bechamp, of Kendall, of Rosenow, of Welch and an army of pleomorphist bacteriologists who would come after him and have to battle the erroneous orthodox laws of Rivers and his legions of followers.

Rife said, "In reality, it is not the bacteria themselves that produce the disease, but the chemical constituents of these micro-organisms enacting upon the unbalanced cell metabolism of the human body that in actuality produce the disease. We also believe if the metabolism of the human body is perfectly balanced or poised, it is susceptible to no disease."

But Rife did not have time to argue theory. He would leave that for others. After isolating the cancer virus, his next step was to destroy it. He did this with his frequency instruments— over and over again. And then he did it with experimental animals, inoculating them, watching the tumors grow, and then killing the virus in their bodies with the same frequency instruments tuned to the same "BX" frequency.

Rife declared in 1953:

"These successful tests were conducted over 400 times with experimental animals before any attempt was made to use this frequency on human cases of carcinoma and sarcoma."

By 1934, Rife was ready to use his frequency instrument on humans. He was ready to cure cancer.

Note: Kendall's "K Medium" was used to grow cancer virus by scientists after the discovery that the virus would grow on it and that ionizing radiation would make the virus more virulent, growing the tumors in weeks instead of months in a spirally wound "argon gas loop" in which the test tubes of the culture would fit for 24 hours at a time. It was made from pig intestine finely desiccated to which a little salt (tyrode solution) was added. Rife discovered that pig meat and mushrooms were a natural cause of cancer in which the cancer virus liked to grow. Rife also discovered the cancer virus in orchids.

Chapter 8
Forward Motion: 1933-1934

Rife had isolated the cancer virus, but a mountain faced him. The filtration versus non-filtration argument prevented those in the field of bacteriology from charging in the direction that Rife, Kendall and Rosenow had shown. Instead, the bacteriologists were squabbling, being skeptical and waiting to see which way the wind blew. The microscope experts also were standing on the sidelines. They had heard or read about the new Rife microscope, but only Rife and Kendall had one, and few knew a second microscope existed in Kendall's Chicago laboratory. Rife wasn't providing the professionals much information. He had his cancer virus to test and test and test. And he had a new, more powerful microscope that he wanted to build. Johnson and others were seeking meetings, writing letters and asking for demonstrations. Rife was polite and helpful at times, but often just never answered his mail. The scientific problem of curing cancer demanded his full attention.

And despite all the outside pressure in 1933, Rife did accomplish three major feats. He wrote a paper which provided a clear direction for future bacteriologists. He continued his cancer research on cultures and guinea pigs—hundreds of them. And he built his new, super microscope.

Rife's brief 1933 paper was titled, "Viruses and Rickettsia of Certain Diseases." A few significant passages are quoted:

"The existing theories regarding the viruses are entirely unsatisfactory and sadly wanting of further elucidation. Therefore, we shall expound our theories at the outset with the hope that other workers may find them sufficiently basic to serve as an incentive for checking our observations.

53

"The writer has long entertained the assumption that it is possible to cultivate viruses on artificial media. . . . The successful results obtained in our initial experiments are on record in a joint publication by Dr. Kendall and myself. . . . The importance of that work was indicated in a later report . . . by E. C. Rosenow, M. D. . . . In this report were recorded the more important observations made during three days, July 5, 6 and 7, 1932 in Dr. Kendall's laboratory at Northwestern University Medical School in Chicago. Assembled there to carry out the experiments were Dr. Kendall, Dr. Rosenow and myself. Owing to the novel and important character of the work, each of us verified at every step the results obtained.

"The above mentioned reports serve to establish two important facts. First that it is possible to culture viruses artificially, and second, that viruses are definitely visible under the Rife Universal Microscope."

The microscope he built in 1933 was the largest and most powerful of the five he built. One was built in 1920, another in 1929, the "Universal" officially completed in 1933 although it may have been used in an uncompleted form in 1932 as the above report suggests, another microscope in 1934, and one in 1937 which was finally finished in 1952. Some parts from pre-existing ones were used for later ones. While the 1929 microscope was a "super" microscope compared to all other commercial microscopes, with a working magnification between 5,000 and 17,000 times, the "Universal" Microscope of 1933 possessed a resolution of 31,000 times and a magnification of 60,000 times (as described in the terms of the time).

An example of the power and clarity of Rife's microscopes compared to other light microscopes is provided by the Smithsonian report of 1944:

"In a recent demonstration of another of the smaller Rife scopes (May 16, 1942) before a group of doctors . . . a Zeiss ruled grating was examined first under an ordinary commercial microscope equipped with a 1.8 high dry lens and × 10 ocular, and then under the Rife microscope. Whereas 50 lines were revealed with the commercial instrument and considerable aberration, both chromatic and spherical noted, only 5 lines were seen with the Rife scope, these 5 lines being so highly magnified that they occupied the entire field, without any aberration whatsoever being apparent. . . . Following the examination of the grating, an ordinary unstained blood film was observed under the same two microscopes. In this instance, 100 cells were seen to spread throughout the field of the commercial instrument while but 10 cells filled the field of the Rife scope."

While Rife was working, so was Dr. Milbank Johnson. Up to this point in time, he seemed to have a minor role—simply putting Rife and Kendall together, sponsoring a dinner, etc. But beginning in 1933, Johnson began to work and organize. He wrote letters. He informed important doctors of what was happening. And he started to plan for the treatment of people who had cancer.

Rife was the pure scientist and undoubtedly a genius of the first order. Milbank Johnson was the political doctor in the best sense of the term. He was a man of the world and an unstoppable executive force. When the scientific honors are finally bestowed on the men who found the cure for cancer and brought it to the world, Dr. Milbank Johnson will be in the first row.

Johnson in the next few years would send Rife numerous letters—informing him, advising him, telling him he was coming to visit and bringing so and so, prodding and subtly pushing Rife. Even if Rife had wanted to avoid Johnson (which he did not), it probably would have been impossible. Johnson was an enormous force of nature—a social energy who, in his own way, was moving mountains.

Johnson's letters indicate that Alvin Foord, the pathologist who later claimed he had little contact with or knowledge of what happened in the 1930s, was in fact deeply and personally involved.

In July 1933, Johnson met Dr. Karl Meyer, the Director of the Hooper Foundation for Medical Research of the University of California in San Francisco. Meyer would later serve on the Special Medical Research Committee of the University of Southern California which sponsored the cancer clinic in 1934 and the other clinics which followed. Years later Meyer would try to claim he had only visited Rife once and looked into his microscopes, not being sure of what he saw. The record clearly indicates a very different situation. In February 1934,

Johnson brought Meyer to San Diego to meet Rife. Johnson later wrote to Rife and Kendall about Meyer's reaction:

To Kendall: "Dr. Meyer was most outspoken in his opinion, using such words as 'conclusive', 'most convincing', 'he is a wizard', and 'he is a genius.'"

To Rife: "You made quite a tremendous impression on Dr. Meyer and I think the whole subject of filtrable bacteria and the microscope were advanced."

In March 1934, Meyer wrote to Rife, "I am still 'dreaming' about the many things you were kind enough to show me last Saturday. As soon as I can tear myself loose I will accept the privilege of coming back and bringing with me some of the agents which produce disease."

In the years to come, the Hooper Foundation would be given a Rife microscope of its own, cancer cultures would be obtained from San Francisco surgeons, and motile colored bodies, "presumably your BX," would be reported to Johnson by Dr. E. L. Walker of the Hooper Foundation, working under Dr. Meyer. Meyer was another non-hero when the AMA and government pressure was imposed. He later served on national medical committees with Dr. Rivers of the Rockefeller Institute and Morris Fishbein of the AMA. But by then he was very silent about the cancer research in which he participated in the 1930s.

In 1933 and 1934, Meyer was one of the growing circle of influential doctors whom Johnson was cultivating as he prepared to organize his credentialed committee to oversee a cancer cure and then bring it to the world.

Johnson was also vigorously defending the filtration theory. When Dr. William J. Robbins of the University of Missouri reported in a *Science News* letter that "one as yet unsettled question about viruses is whether or not they actually are living organisms," Johnson wrote to him and referred him to the articles by Kendall, Rife and Rosenow. He also put himself on record:

"I have seen with Dr. Karl Meyer of the University of California the filter passing forms of such diseases as hog cholera, psittacosis, and a very infectious disease of chickens

56

affecting their throat. . . . It seems strange to me that others are having difficulty first—in producing the filter passing organisms; and second—that there should be the least doubt about their existence, form, characteristics, or size when they are so easy to obtain and so easy to determine. . . . I feel quite sure that Dr. Kendall in Chicago who has the Rife microscope nearest to you will verify what I have said and show you these for yourself."

But while Johnson was willing to serve as a frontline soldier in the filtration war, his true role was as a general in the cancer war. In the Spring of 1934, he rented the "ranch" of a member of the famous Scripps family of the Scripps Oceanographic Institute. The ranch in La Jolla outside San Diego was to be used as a clinic for the first treatment of cancer victims using the Rife Frequency Instrument.

Johnson was moving, pushing and manipulating. He wrote to Kendall on April 2, 1934, "I hope you and Gertrude will be able to spend your vacation in La Jolla this year. . . . It is going to take all the ingenuity of a Rife and Kendall plus the little help that a poor M.D. like myself can give before we are going to be able to crack this nut. But we are going to crack it if we have to drop it from a height of ten miles."

Then Johnson exposed his own driving motive:

"You don't know how hard it is for me to keep my shirt on in this whole proposition because I can't help but see in my mind's eye the tens of thousands of discouraged, hopeless, suffering individuals dying by inches with cancer who might be saved. Of course I know that you and Rife are interested in this thing from a pure science standpoint, but unfortunately, my training has been largely mixed with the humanities and it is real sickening to see the suffering and hopelessness of the victims of this terrible disease."

At the same time, Johnson began "prepping" Rife for the upcoming clinic. On the second page of a letter to Rife in early April 1934, just a few months before the cancer clinic was to get underway, Johnson wrote what may become an immortal scientific paragraph:

"Incidentally, I am thinking about taking a house in La Jolla from June 15 to September 15. If by that time you get far

57

enough along in your work, I would like to try your method on a human being or so."

On April 30, 1934, Johnson again wrote to Rife:

"Can't you meet me about 11:30 in La Jolla next Saturday. I want to show you the Library Building and get your opinion of it before I say anything to the people at the Scripps Clinic about it as a place for our Clinic this Summer."

Chapter 9

The Cancer Cure Works!

The full story of the cancer clinic of 1934 may never be known. Rife's records were lost when he foolishly loaned them to Dr. Arthur Yale a few years later. Yale had started his own clinic and apparently wanted to compare notes. After Rife learned that Dr. Yale was altering the Frequency Instrument and thus failing to get results, Rife and Yale had an argument which marked a permanent separation. More disturbing is that after AMA pressure forced a law suit against the production company making the Frequency Instruments, many of the doctors who were involved became exceedingly cautious. And after Milbank Johnson's death, the records at the University of Southern California "mysteriously disappeared."

But pieces of evidence do exist and while the clinical records are gone, there is sufficient documentation to know that astounding results did take place and that the Special Medical Research Committee did continue to exist. The listings under the name of Milbank Johnson in *Who's Who* for 1944-45 (Johnson died October 3, 1944) include:

"Professor physiology and clinical medicine, University of Southern California 1897-1901, *now* Chairman special medical research committee of the university."

Until Johnson's death in 1944, he was still actively the head of the committee. For 10 years from its creation in 1934, Johnson's University of Southern California Medical Research Committee was in existence. Given the fact that testimonials exist describing what occurred and that Johnson ran his own clinic from 1935 to 1938, there is no reason to believe—as later was implied by the AMA and the California State Public

59

Health agency—that the existence of a successful cancer cure in 1934 using the Frequency Instrument was a myth. Documents show the clinic existed and succeeded in curing cancer. And doctors who continued treating seriously ill people with success because of what the Frequency Instrument accomplished in 1934 tell the real story, as do the signed reports from cured cancer patients in later years.

Johnson eventually handed his authority over to Dr. James Couche of San Diego. Couche was not a heavyweight in California medical circles as was Johnson. It was a poor choice if the goal was to move the medical profession toward acceptance and widespread use of Rife's new healing technology. The result was total failure. But Couche was the right choice if the standard was to choose a man who would not quit or knuckle under to the AMA. Couche used the Frequency Instrument for 22 years and reported for the record—if only briefly—on his continued success with a Frequency Instrument that stayed calibrated as Rife insisted it had to be if it was to destroy the pathologic micro-organisms in people.

But all that lay ahead. In the summer of 1934, 16 terminally ill people with cancer and other diseases were brought to the Scripps "ranch." There, as Rife and the doctors worked on human beings for the first time, they learned much. The early patients were exposed to the frequency for only 3 minutes, but Rife soon learned that if a treatment was given every day, the toxins from the dead micro-organisms accumulated faster than the body could dispose of them. When he switched to a treatment of 3 minutes every 3rd day, the patients began healing swiftly.

In 1953 when Rife copyrighted his book, he made the real report of what happened in 1934. Anyone who has examined his life, his patience, his scientific commitment, and the correctness of his filtration studies (which are now being verified by bacteriologists who never heard his name) must consider that his own scientific report of the 1934 cancer clinic carries some weight. He wrote:

"With the frequency instrument treatment, no tissue is destroyed, no pain is felt, no noise is audible, and no sensation is noticed. A tube lights up and 3 minutes later the treatment is completed. The virus or bacteria is destroyed and the body then recovers itself naturally from the toxic effect of the virus or bacteria. Several diseases may be treated simultaneously.

"The first clinical work on cancer was completed under the supervision of Milbank Johnson, M.D. which was set up under a Special Medical Research Committee of the University of Southern California. 16 cases were treated at the clinic for many types of malignancy. After 3 months, 14 of these so-called hopeless cases were signed off as clinically cured by the staff of five medical doctors and Dr. Alvin G. Foord, M.D. Pathologist for the group. The treatments consisted of 3 minutes duration using the frequency instrument which was set on the mortal oscillatory rate for 'BX' or cancer (at 3 day intervals). It was found that the elapsed time between treatments attains better results than the cases treated daily. This gives the lymphatic system an opportunity to absorb and cast off the toxic condition which is produced by the devitalized dead particles of the 'BX' virus. No rise of body temperature was perceptible in any of these cases above normal during or after the frequency instrument treatment. No special diets were used in any of this clinical work, but we sincerely believe that a proper diet compiled for the individual would be of benefit."

Date: December 1, 1953
Written by R. R. Rife

Other members of the clinic were Whalen Morrison, Chief Surgeon of the Santa Fe Railway, George C. Dock, M.D., internationally famous, George C. Fischer, M.D., Children's Hospital in New York, Arthur I. Kendall, Dr. Zite, M.D., professor of pathology at Chicago University, Rufus B. Von Klein Schmidt, President of the University of Southern California.

Dr. Couche and Dr. Carl Meyer, Ph.D., head of the Department of Bacteriological Research at the Hooper Foundation in San Francisco were also present. Dr. Kopps of the Metabolic Clinic in La Jolla signed all 14 reports and knew of all the tests from his personal observation.

A week after the clinic ended, Kendall wrote to Mrs. Bridges, wife of Rife's original sponsor:

"This afternoon (September 20, 1934) I have a meeting with Mr. Hardin, President of the Board of Trustees of the

University; he is much interested in Roy and his splendid work, and I shall be asked to tell what I saw during my very brief visit to California. Mr. Hardin, unlike many persons, is very friendly, and will take the proper view of the work: that it is experimental so far, done with no rules of the game to go by, and with a machine that is designed for small output, and therefore, not capable of showing its full worth. I understand there is to be a new machine, embodying the facts learned from the old one, and built along more lusty lines so its output will be more nearly equal to the demands which should be put upon it. I have written to Dr. Johnson telling him about the one case I can talk intelligently about: Tom Knight. Roy will tell you about Tom: he seems to me to be the most important case of the entire series because his tumor was on the cheek, where it could be seen, watched and measured from the start to the finish. This I have done, reciting the actual measurements, and details of treatment and of pathological examination."

One year later on September 18, 1935, Milbank Johnson wrote to Dr. Thomas Burger and Dr. C. Ray Launsberry of San Diego:

"This will introduce to you Mr. Thomas Knight. He was the man who had the carcinoma over the malar bone of his left cheek that we treated at the clinic in La Jolla last year."

In 1956, Dr. James Couche made the following declaration:

"I would like to make this historical record of the amazing scientific wonders regarding the efficacy of the frequencies of the Royal R. Rife Frequency Instrument. . . .

"When I was told about Dr. Rife and his frequency instrument at the Ellen Scripps home near the Scripps Institute Annex some twenty-two years ago, I went out to see about it and became very interested in the cases which he had there. And the thing that brought me into it more quickly than anything was a man who had a cancer of the stomach. Rife was associated at that time with Dr. Milbank Johnson, M.D., who was then president of the Medical Association of Los Angeles, a very wealthy man and a very big man in the medical world— the biggest in Los Angeles and he had hired this annex for this demonstration over a summer of time.

"In that period of time I saw many things and the one that impressed me the most was a man who staggered onto a table, just on the last end of cancer; he was a bag of bones. As he lay on the table, Dr. Rife and Dr. Johnson said, 'Just feel that man's stomach.' So I put my hand on the cavity where his stomach was underneath and it was just a cavity almost, because he was so thin; his backbone and his belly were just about touching each other.

"I put my hand on his stomach which was just one solid mass, just about what I could cover with my hand, somewhat like the shape of a heart. It was absolutely solid! And I thought to myself, well, nothing can be done for that. However, they gave him a treatment with the Rife frequencies and in the course of time over a period of six weeks to two months, to my astonishment, he completely recovered. He got so well that he asked permission to go to El Centro as he had a farm there and he wanted to see about his stock. Dr. Rife said, 'Now you haven't the strength to drive to El Centro.'

"'Oh, yes' said he. 'I have, but I'll have a man to drive me there.' As a matter of fact, the patient drove his own car there and when he got down to El Centro he had a sick cow and he stayed up all night with it. The next day he drove back without any rest whatsoever—so you can imagine how he had recovered.

"I saw other cases that were very interesting. Then I wanted a copy of the frequency instrument. I finally bought one of these frequency instruments and established it in my office.

"I saw some very remarkable things resulting from it in the course of over twenty years.

"I had a Mexican boy, nine years of age, who had osteomyelitis of the leg. He was treated at the Mercy Hospital by his attending doctors. They scraped the bone every week. It was agonizing to the child because they never gave him anything; they just poked in there and cleaned him out and the terror of that boy was awful. He wore a splint and was on crutches. His family brought him to the office. He was terrified that I would poke him as the other doctors had done. I reassured him and demonstrated the instrument on my own hand to show him that it would not hurt. With the bandage and splint still on he was given a treatment. In less than two weeks of treatment the wound was completely healed and he took off his splints and threw them away. He is a great big powerful man now and has never had any comeback of his osteomyelitis. He was completely cured. There were many cases such as this."

63

In December 1935, Dr. Johnson wrote a confidential letter to Dr. Mildred Schram, Secretary of the International Cancer Research Foundation in Philadelphia. In that letter, Johnson explained why the records of the 1934 cancer clinic were sketchy:

> "The clinic was opened and run by me to satisfy me personally whether the Rife Ray would destroy pathogenic organisms in vivo as well as in vitro. The latter we had repeatedly demonstrated in the laboratory. I had to have this information conclusively positive before I could recommend to my friends to get in behind the work to carry it to a logical conclusion. Having no nurses or secretaries in La Jolla, the records, while truthful, are more or less fragmentary and not kept for careful scrutiny by brother scientists. As I told you, when I started this work I intended to finance it through to the end. The only assistance that I expected to get was such cooperation as I might receive from other physicians in working with the Microscope and the Ray.
>
> "Now that we have to convince a whole lot of other men from cold turkey, we shall have to turn over a new leaf and do our work subject to inspection by others."

So the success story of 1934, while true as attested by Rife's written record, Couche's story of the incredible recovery by the farmer, and Kendall-Johnson's correspondence on the man with the neck tumor, also was unsatisfactory in terms of providing documented medical reports for other scientists. The 1934 clinic was a first, tentative, experimental step. They learned that treatment was best given every third day. They realized that they would have to keep better records. They recognized that the Frequency Instrument would have to be improved.

But they did cure cancer. And when it is realized how quickly radiation therapy was financed and the machines put into hospitals (with such meager results), the tragedy of not being able to finance mass production of Rife's Frequency Instrument can be appreciated in its full horror.

If Milbank Johnson was wracked by the thought of tens of thousands suffering in the 1930s, he'd be staggered by the 460,000 Americans now dying every year and the 900,000 Americans every year who learn that they have cancer. And he'd be broken by the sight of "treatment" with chemotherapy, radiation and surgery. As Rife had shown, the cancer BX changed form. If all its forms weren't destroyed, the cancer micro-organism could find another environment in a weakened body and start anew. The tragic legacy of the Bechamp failure with Pasteur and the Rife-Kendall failure with Rivers would come back to haunt humanity with a grim vengeance.

Chapter 10
1935: Climbing A Mountain

In a letter dated October 15, 1935, Dr. Milbank Johnson explained to a cancer foundation why Rife and he couldn't stop their work and do special tests which the foundation wanted:

"From what I have said I don't want you to jump to the conclusion that we are not interested in your side of the problem because we are, but with the limited means at our disposal we don't like to break into our planned procedure at this most interesting juncture of the work. You know in mountain climbing better progress is made to keep going up and up all the time. If you stop and go back every once in awhile, you are very apt to wear yourself out and waste your energies and never reach the top. This is about all I can say until I have discussed the matter fully with Mr. Rife."

Indeed 1935 was a year of mountain climbing. Rife built new, more accurate frequency instruments. He began planning a new laboratory. He built a smaller microscope which could be mass produced. Research continued. The second clinic was opened. Visitors came—a well-known cancer expert, a representative from the cancer foundation, an associate of Dr. Meyer at the Hooper Foundation in San Francisco who had to be trained so that the Rife experiments could be independently verified.

And always there was pressure to announce the findings. Newall Jones of the San Diego *Evening Tribune* had written Rife a letter in September 1934 and talked to him on the telephone after Jones discovered what was going on at the 1934 cancer clinic. He promised to handle the story carefully and, with Rife, to plan the story in advance. Jones fully understood the significance of what Rife was doing. Jones:

"If your research comes to a successful conclusion, it would not only constitute a remarkable contribution to medicine and science—that goes without saying—but, because of its importance to all humanity, would quite naturally be a great news story. Naturally, we would like to get that story."

Jones would have to wait three and a half years, but in May 1938 he would write the clearest explanations of the Rife discoveries which would ever appear in a newspaper.

In early March 1935, Johnson received a letter from the International Cancer Research Foundation in Philadelphia. There were many questions they wanted answered, plus photographs of the laboratory, and photographs of the microscope. From this communication began a series of exchanges, proposals and visits which ultimately produced nothing. In retrospect, part of the failure can be seen as simple human misunderstanding, but the time wasted over the next year and a half can also be judged as the fault of pettiness, arrogance and narrow-minded obstinacy on the part of the International Cancer Research Foundation, particularly its rigid Secretary, Dr. Mildred Schram. The Foundation was in a position to fund Rife in such a way that major advances could have quickly resulted. Instead, they argued for tests which were not relevant. They wasted Rife's time by having him make a demonstration in Philadelphia the next year, and then they failed to keep their agreement on the techniques he showed them, instead insisting on their own—which ruined the procedure. In their example also lies one of the dilemmas of modern research. The experts have their own way of doing things. The great scientist who is an outsider is looked down upon by the "authorities"—those with the "credentials." The goal of curing cancer becomes secondary. The existing procedures take precedence.

In the exchanges between Johnson and the International Cancer Research Foundation can be seen the institutional strait jackets which also bind modern scientists. With 460,000 Americans dying of cancer every year, the widest variety of cancer treatments should be encouraged. Unfortunately, such a program would encroach on the territory and the financial income of the established "experts."

By June 1935 the International Cancer Foundation reported to Johnson that four insurance companies were interested in financing Rife if the foundation gave its approval. The foundation asked to send its representative to visit Rife's laboratory.

Dr. Mildred Schram, Secretary of the Foundation, arrived at the end of July 1935, but it was a hurried visit because of her other West Coast commitments. Johnson wrote back to her in September: "The next time you come I hope you will not be loaded down with any other duties so that you can give your undivided attention to our work. Dr. Walker, who is an expert in his line, spent three weeks familiarizing himself with our technique and the microscope, so, in the short time you had it was impossible for you to get more than a smattering idea of what we are driving at."

Schram replied that she expected Rife to cultivate and identify the causes of the disease in mice she had shipped to Rife. It was as if they were to pass an examination! Johnson wrote back that they were completing the new frequency instruments, had focused for years on the cancer virus in humans and couldn't be expected to undertake the kind of work the foundation expected—identifying the cancer micro-organisms in different mice. Johnson declared:

"Trying to cultivate strange germs and identify them in malignant tissue is just about as difficult and tedious a job as one can undertake and does not want interruption if a worthwhile job is to be done. We could not at that particular time have followed out your instructions and desires even if we had understood them."

But William H. Donner, President of the International Cancer Research Foundation, had become "deeply interested" in Rife and his discoveries. So Schram stayed in contact. Nevertheless, she insisted on the test she had designed.

In mid-October 1935, Johnson tried again to explain:

"I don't think you can really appreciate what it means to culture three unknown organisms, if there are that many, ascertain the M.O.R. (Mortal Oscillatory Rate) for each of them, and later on to take a series of animals and attempt to destroy that organism. As you know, our work thus far has been devoted exclusively to human cancer, and a single organism which we have found up to this time always present in human cancer has taken a tremendous lot of time already to study the life history and the life cycle of that one. I am not sure that Mr. Rife or our Committee would wish to drop that work and undertake this much larger problem of studying the different hyperplasias and tumors that might occur in different strains of mice which may or may not have a relation to human carcinoma."

Johnson suggested that the foundation President William Donner take his winter vacation in San Diego instead of Bermuda or Florida. But Donner was neither a doctor nor a bacteriologist. He was a steel executive, bank trustee and corporate mogul. Schram was the professional power at the foundation. She wrote back immediately stating her tests were necessary if the foundation was to put up any money. She insisted that they do the tests as she specified.

In December 1935, Schram informed Johnson that action had been deferred on his grant request. But she relented on her test. The possibilities of Rife's cure were too important to dismiss on her personal whim, especially when so many experts—bacteriologists, doctors and microscopists—were talking about Rife's work. So, instead of her test, she asked for detailed information on the cancer clinic of 1934, insisting that the well-known Dr. Dock of Johnson's Special Research Committee provide it. If the material provided was sufficient, she indicated, a grant might be forthcoming. She then also admitted that her tests really weren't necessary once the research grant was bestowed. They had been required previously only to get the grant! Exactly 9 months had passed, most of that time wasted because of Schram's narrow-minded insistence on a procedure of her design.

Johnson's exasperation showed in his reply. He explained the kind of clinical records that did exist and pushed for a simpler solution—a foundation representative in Rife's laboratory for a few weeks. Johnson:

"You are right in protecting your funds from waste. But, I still think that a properly qualified scientist or clinician could learn more in two weeks by actually trying the things himself than he can learn by correspondence in a year."

Nevertheless, Johnson did manage to get Rife to describe the Frequency Instrument and he did call a meeting of the Special Medical Research Committee of the University of Southern California. Dr. Dock would be leaving a week later for a trip around the world, so it is assumed that some statement of the full committee, including Dock, was Johnson's goal—in order that the foundation could have a basis for a grant. However, after another year of correspondence and meetings, nothing would come of the effort.

The interaction with the International Cancer Research Institute was only one element of Johnson's and Rife's "mountain climb" in 1935. Far more important was the visit from O. Cameron Gruner, a well-known cancer researcher from Montreal. Gruner would bring his own discovery just as Kendall had done in 1931, and Rife would take Gruner's discovery and join it with Kendall's and his own. The result would be another breakthrough.

Gruner had taken blood from his cancer patients and from it, on an Asparagus Medium, had grown a fungus. Rife put Dr. Gruner's fungus in the "K Medium" and then filtered from it Rife's own "BX" virus. He then put some of his earlier BX on Gruner's Asparagus Medium and brought forth Gruner's fungus. Another form of the cancer micro-organism had been isolated—a fungus!

Rife now had a solid base for *pleomorphism*. Not only could the BX virus live on an artificial medium, but the BX could change into another form in the blood (the monococcoid form in the monocytes of the blood of over 90% of cancer patients) and then into still another form—a crytomyces pleomorphia fungus.

Rife conclusively stated in his 1953 report: "This BX virus can be readily changed into different forms of its life cycle by the media upon which it is grown."

In 1937, Milbank Johnson wrote a letter describing what Dr. Gruner and Royal Rife had discovered in May-June 1935:

"Dr. Gruner was present at all the experiments and we agreed—I think beyond a doubt—that our BX and the organism which he obtained from the blood, although in a different form from our BX, are one and the same organism. It looks, there-

71

fore, as if we know how to produce at will, by means of the appropriate culture, any one of the three forms desired."

Dr. Schram at the International Cancer Research Institute was informed of this discovery. Part of the proposed grant was to be used to bring Dr. Gruner to San Diego for a year to work alongside Rife. Schram referred in one letter to the "Gruner-Johnson-Rife organism." In light of Dr. Gruner's reputation in cancer research and the discovery resulting from his experiments with Rife, Schram's prolonged insistence on a test of her design, which she later admitted was not central to the grant, demonstrates how the "system" then and today often operates: on the basis of personal priorities disguised as professional requirements.

In May 1935, Johnson also began looking for a location in Los Angeles for a new clinic. It presented a bit of a problem because the electric current had to be 60 cycles for the new Frequency Instrument. Finally the Santa Fe Hospital at 610 South Saint Louis Street on a corner with East Sixth Street in Los Angeles was chosen. The clinic opened the first week of November 1935 with Johnson in charge. Treatments were given two days a week, and this time Johnson was keeping careful clinical records.

The new Frequency Instrument was finished in September 1935. Rife, his new assistant Philip Hoyland, his earlier assistant Jack Free, and Milbank Johnson then put the new machine into operation. Johnson explained the process:

> "The new Rife Ray Machine had arrived at its point of construction when elaborate tests had to be made in order to synchronize the M.O.R. produced by it with the M.O.R. produced by the old machine. Now, we are in the throes of accurately charting the 14,000 possible settings on the new machine. Our next process, beginning next week, is to test its penetration, the time required in the different exposures, the different depths of lesions. So, take it altogether we are just about as busy as a bear in berrytime."

Later that year, Rife provided a brief description of the Frequency Instrument, presumably because of the Foundation's request:

> "The basic principle of this device is the control of a desired

72

frequency. These frequencies varying upon the organism being treated.

"The frequency is set which controls the initial oscillator, which in turn is run through six stages of amplification, the last stage driving a 50 watt output tube.

"The frequency with its carrier wave is transmitted into an output tube similar to the standard X ray tube, but filled with a different inert gas. This tube acts as a directional antenna.

"The importance in the variable control of these frequencies is that each pathogenic organism being treated is of a different chemical constituency, the consequence being they carry a different molecular vibratory rate. Each one in turn under these conditions requires a different frequency or vibratory rate to destroy."

The new instrument was light-socket powered and had an output of 500 watts. Furthermore, it was equipped to deliver two distinct frequencies simultaneously and both variable. This apparatus proved to be more efficient with decidedly fewer factors of error.

Rife also—amazing as it seems given everything else occurring in his life—built a new, smaller microscope. While the "Universal" microscope of 1933 cost between $30,000-$35,000 to construct, according to Johnson, the 1935 microscope was theoretically priced to be sold at $1,000 or less. The purpose was to make many of the smaller microscopes available to research laboratories. The new microscope still had a magnification range of 10,000 times to 15,000 times— far beyond what the "best" light microscopes available could do.

Then there was Dr. Walker's visit of three weeks. This occurred in August after his boss, Dr. Karl Meyer, had established the training session when Meyer visited Rife on June 28, 1935. Walker learned about the laboratory procedures, about the "BX" virus (carcinoma), about the "BY" virus (sarcoma), and about the Rife microscope. He then returned to San Francisco to work with Dr. Karl Meyer at the Hooper Foundation. Later, he was provided a Rife microscope of his own.

In October 1935, Dr. Walker wrote:

"The copy of the results of your test of the Rife ray on

typhoid organisms would appear to establish conclusively the efficiency of it to kill these organisms in the tissues. If the ray should prove equally efficient in killing other pathogenic micro-organisms, it would be the greatest discovery in the history of therapeutic medicine."

Walker soon found that his work would be far more difficult than he originally envisioned. He eventually would isolate a BX on his own with old antiquated equipment provided by Rife, but not before he experienced shock at the lack of support he received from his colleagues. One of his letters in late 1935 referred to his being held up by a mercenary person. Another letter tells how the surgeons in San Francisco wouldn't cooperate—they wouldn't provide any cancer tissues!

And throughout 1935, Johnson was keeping an eye on some of the patients from the 1934 cancer clinic. In May he wrote Rife and asked him to visit Tom Knight, the patient whose healing had so impressed Arthur Kendall and whose tumor Kendall had measured so carefully. Johnson to Rife: "You will find Tom's address on your copy of his case record. I want you to have a look at old Tom yourself and see whether there is any recurrence of the cancer, either on the face or in the glands, also, look at his lip."

In October, Johnson wrote Rife's assistant to look up the M.O.R. for the disease they treated in another 1934 patient, Wayne Grayson. Johnson explained he had the man's clinical record, but he had failed to record the M.O.R. at the time of treatment.

As the year ended, the Special Medical Research Committee of the University of Southern California met to analyze the progress. The meeting was held on December 26 in Los Angeles.

And indeed the progress of 1936 was phenomenal—a new Frequency Instrument, a new microscope, a second clinic underway, the historic discovery with Dr. Gruner of Montreal, the training of Dr. Walker of San Francisco. Only the fiasco with the International Cancer Research Foundation marred the "going up and up all the time" as Rife, Johnson and their gathering band attacked the mountain.

Chapter 11
1936: "Astounding" Clinic Results

Sometime in early 1936 William Donner, the President of the International Cancer Research Foundation, visited Rife and Johnson. He was impressed by what he saw and wanted his colleagues in Philadelphia to witness a demonstration. Rife agreed to travel east in the spring and show them how to filter a BX cancer virus.

Also in early 1936, Johnson and Henry Timken, Rife's original sponsor, completed agreements to build the wonderful laboratory Rife had so long envisioned. The ground was broken in April and Rife moved in during the latter part of July.

Rife and Philip Hoyland began revising the Frequency Instrument in the early months of 1936, eliminating parts which had been made obsolete by recent advances in electronics. During that summer they produced an entirely new method of generating the desired frequencies. Among the new test appliances they created was a nine inch Cathode-Ray oscillograph of high sensitivity, built for the purpose of photographing the different frequencies on motion picture film. This enabled them to study and classify the numerous waves in an entirely new way.

In April Rife traveled to San Francisco to help Dr. Walker get his test procedures refined. On May 1, he left for Chicago where he attended an electronics convention. From there he traveled to Louisville where an eye doctor examined him and restricted his daily use of the microscope to two hours. On May 9, 1936, he arrived in Philadelphia for the fateful meeting with the International Cancer Research Foundation. What followed belongs in the category of tragic fiascos.

In February of the next year, Johnson wrote to Dr. Edward

Archibald, Canada's most renowned cancer specialist and an associate of Dr. Gruner who had collaborated with Rife in the Spring of 1935. Johnson described to Dr. Archibald what Rife encountered in Philadelphia during his May 1936 demonstration:

> "Rife reported that they provided him with six or seven tumors without any pathological report whatsoever on any of them. He examined them microscopically and found that all but three had been heavily rayed with X-ray or had been treated with radium. The three which had not been treated, he planted and irradiated in the argon tube in accordance with our technique. In each case, he obtained the characteristic BX. They insisted upon keeping some of the material so obtained and said they were going to try to produce cancers in animals of their own. We have never been notified whether or not they did so. The atmosphere in which Mr. Rife found himself was one of extreme skepticism. They were urged not to try to reproduce these experiments without first learning our techniques by actual experience, but were determined to go ahead, and if they did so, they probably failed."

On May 22, 1936, William Donner wrote to Johnson and told him no grant would be forthcoming for at least 100 days or so, thereby breaking the promise he had given Johnson and Rife at the beginning of the year. Johnson's reply on May 27 is an anguished plea for the Foundation to finance Dr. Gruner for a period of time at Rife's side in San Diego instead of paying an inexperienced clinician in Philadelphia to try replicating Rife's procedures. The plea fell on deaf ears, but is worth quoting at some length. It exemplifies how one man's clear thinking (in this case Johnson's) may be more important in accomplishing a research goal than all the prestige, careful procedures and credentialed expertise that an important foundation can organize. Johnson wrote:

> "Your letter came as a great disappointment to me. I had thought from what you told me in the winter, that we might hope for an immediate grant if Mr. Rife was able to show to your man the BX taken from human carcinoma and the method by which the organism was grown.
> "I understood you to say that you felt so strongly about it that if Mr. Rife were successful, you yourself would be willing

76

to give Dr. Gruner's services for a year if your Board, which did not believe in the bacterial origin of cancer, was unwilling to make the grant.

"You secured Dr. Dodge who, I agree, is one of the finest mycologists in America. He worked every minute, step by step, with Mr. Rife. Notes were taken of every detail of each day's work, and these notes were signed daily by both Dr. Dodge and Mr. Rife. This shows how entirely frank Mr. Rife was in showing every minute step of the process to Dr. Dodge.

"As this same organism has been repeatedly found by us and also by Dr. Arthur I. Kendall in Chicago, and now in Philadelphia, you and your board can surely assume that if not the sole cause of cancer, it is at least constantly present in that disease. So far as we know, no other research group has gone so far.

"A delay until October is almost tragic at this stage of the work. Dr. Gruner has had invitations to go elsewhere, but has waited to see if we could secure the grant to carry on the work, as he believes we are further along than any other research group.

"In delaying until October, are you not demanding from us more than from a research organization? We cannot *prove* these points without further research and we have always understood that the organizations to which you have already given grants are merely research organizations.

"You say that you are selecting a man in Philadelphia to carry on the inoculating and the growing of the organisms from human cancer during Dr. Dodge's absence. Perhaps you do not realize that it is impossible to handle filter-passing forms of bacteria without a microscope which shows them. Only by this means can the work be properly checked from day to day.

"As you undoubtedly must pay the man whom you select in Philadelphia to do this work, would you not be willing to employ Dr. Gruner yourself to work out here with Mr. Rife and his microscope? He would have every facility and every probability of success.

"May I remind you that over three years ago, Dr. Arthur I. Kendall of Northwestern Medical School published his epochal work on filter-passing organisms, and that since that time, many, many scientists have tried in vain to repeat his experiments. Such men as Park of New York, and Zinsser of Harvard, having failed in their attempts, have vociferously

77

denied the existence of these filter-passing organisms. You yourself know how mistaken that is.

"We have found no way to grow these organisms except in the Kendall medium, and even when Kendall medium has been supplied to these other scientists, they have not been able to sterilize the medium without ruining it.

"It would seem to me, in view of these facts and the peculiar situation in which this matter seems to be involved, that it would be wise to select someone in whom you have every confidence and send him to the Rife Laboratory to work this problem out. Do you not feel that it should be someone who has actually grown filter-passing organisms and can see and recognize them? If you are unwilling to give us Dr. Gruner, will you not send a man whom you have selected here to us?

"I cannot believe that any man lacking experience in handling filter-passing organisms and without a Rife microscope can succeed in many times the 100 days which you cite as a minimum.

"You and we are seeking to conquer this horrible human curse. I realize that the general acceptance of our views will completely revolutionize present concepts concerning the causes of many diseases besides cancer. Therefore, the greatest care must be taken in each step if we are to avoid at least some of the tremendous antagonisms which always greet new ideas. For that reason, we are willing to go to extremes in checking our findings and having them checked, but we do *not* want to be checked by inexperienced men in a matter involving so highly technical and so specialised a knowledge.

"Hoping you will bear with me and will consider patiently each point which this letter has tried to bring before you, I am

Very seriously yours,
Milbank Johnson"

On June 2, 1936, William Donner turned down Milbank Johnson's plea. The International Cancer Research Institute would do their own tests. At the end of September, Mildred Schram wrote to Rife, asking for his advice as they completed their experiments. In October, Donner wrote to Rife. Rife refused to answer them. In November, Donner telegraphed Johnson. Then wrote him again. But Rife had wasted enough time with them. He was curing cancer while the foundation broke their agreements, insisted on procedures with inexperienced people which were doomed from the outset, and ignored the larger goal which Rife was achieving—the cure of cancer in human beings.

Sometime in the spring of 1936, Johnson closed his clinic at the Santa Fe Hospital. The results had been impressive, but he wanted to pause because of the improvements being made in the Frequency Instrument and then open the third clinic in the fall of 1936.

On April 28, 1936, Dr. Harry Goodman, an eye specialist, wrote to Johnson describing the effect of the Frequency Instrument on Mrs. Julia M. Gowdy. She had been examined previously on March 23. A little more than a month later, her vision had improved 29% in one eye and 10% in the other. "It had been difficult for her to read the telephone book but now she gets the numbers rather quickly," Goodman reported.

In September, Dr. James Couche of San Diego, who had witnessed the first cancer clinic at the Scripps Ranch in 1934, began conducting a clinic with the help of Jack Free, Rife's assistant. They treated cancer and senile cataracts. While the records are incomplete, the first three were cancer patients and according to Couche's notes, all completely recovered.

Also in September, Dr. Milbank Johnson opened his third clinic in the Pasadena Home for the Aged. The clinic lasted until May 1937. Johnson's description of his success and the incredible medical events he was witnessing were preserved in copies of letters he sent to Dr. Gruner in Canada and to Dr. Meyer in San Francisco just before the year ended.

To Gruner, Johnson wrote, "The clinic is held three mornings a week, Tuesday, Thursday and Saturday. Yesterday I had eighteen patients. Among them were two cases of pulmonary tuberculosis, three cases of carcinoma, two cases of chronic varicose ulcers of the leg, and sundry other cases of more or less definite infection origin. . . . I certainly wish you were here to work with me because I am afraid that even you, who know what we are trying to do, will not believe some of the yarns that I would have to tell you as to what is occurring in that clinic without actually seeing them yourself."

To Dr. Meyer, Johnson reported:

"At times the results of the Ray are absolutely astounding,

causing an instantaneous sterilization of the wounds, whether interior or exterior."

The Special Medical Research Committee was still in charge however and they were keeping a tight clamp on any announcement until the procedures were certain. In April 1936, prior to Rife's Philadelphia visit, Johnson had specifically instructed Donner that everything the foundation witnessed was to be held in strict confidence. Johnson insisted that "there should be no publication nor any kind of publicity attending this demonstration without the consent of the Special Medical Research Committee of the University of Southern California. We are doing this to prevent any premature publication and the raising of false hopes before things have been thoroughly proven."

In early December, Johnson wrote to Meyers asking when he could be in Los Angeles in order that Johnson could schedule a meeting of the Committee. There was much to report.

And then, ten days before Christmas, Johnson and Rife got a Christmas present from San Francisco. Dr. E. L. Walker, Meyer's coworker at the Hooper Foundation, had (on his own, independent of Rife) isolated in June 1936 the *fungus* form of cancer—crytomyces pleomorphia. In December, he announced he had isolated from a cancer breast the virus form—"motile colored bodies under the Rife microscope, presumably your BX."

Chapter 12

1937: Money Woes and Delays

1937 was a year of frustration. Johnson and Rife were trying to get Dr. Gruner from Montreal to join Rife in his laboratory. The Special Research Committee of the University of Southern California was hoping to make an announcement by the end of the year concerning the "etiology of cancer." It was decided that they would announce only how cancer developed—how the virus changed form. They were not going to tell the public about the treatment. They knew that there would be tremendous scientific opposition when they described how cancer developed and why other researchers hadn't been able to isolate the "germ." So they reasoned that they had to establish cancer's etiology before announcing the unique Frequency Instrument cure.

Yet, given what they knew, the clinical records that they had, and the microscope's capacity to disprove the claims of the opposition, their caution was undoubtedly one of the worst decisions they ever made. They were naïve about the financial, scientific, and medical opposition as well as how the Rife discoveries would threaten these powerful interests. Within a few years, they would discover to what lengths the men at the top of these three professions would go to crush them and suppress the cure for cancer. But in 1937, they thought that they could be conservative. They believed that conservatism would advance their goal. It was a deadly error, for almost 50 years would pass before the American public finally learned about Rife's scientific miracle.

Dr. George Dock, the internationally famous member of the Special Research Committee, was now working actively with Johnson to interest other prominent men in the Committee's work. He would later side with the AMA, keeping quiet about the suppression and accepting the AMA's highest award, but in 1937 he joined Johnson in the front lines.

In late December 1936 and early 1937, Dr. Johnson and Dr. Dock had long converstions with Dr. Charles Martin, former Dean of McGill University in Montreal. Their purpose was to convince him that Dr. Gruner had to join Rife. Martin returned to Canada after his talks with Johnson and Dock. There Martin attempted to have McGill University pay for Gruner to work for several months in the Rife Laboratory. But Martin failed. The Depression went into a frightening second stage in 1937-38. Money was limited. And those in Montreal who were opposed to Gruner's findings were not willing to support financially a project which could result in even more findings to their dislike. Gruner later was assigned two laboratory associates who were convinced "monomorphists." Thus, his work in proving pleomorphism and particularly the cancer etiology was obstructed, if not actually sabotaged.

It is important to recognize that many of the men involved in the Rife work were doctors and researchers. They were not men who fought political battles and in many ways they crumbled when they were challenged by determined political power. They believed in scientific procedures. Even today in the mid-1980s, men and women of similar good will and naïveté conduct the research procedures. In discussing the Rife cancer cure with such people, it is common to hear top men in physics, microscopy and cancer research state, "Suppression of a cancer cure in the 1930s is impossible. Scientists would have known about it. It couldn't be covered up." The truth is that the cure for cancer *was* covered up. And the naïveté of cancer researchers as well as scientists in related fields persists to modern times.

The question now is, what will they do when they learn the facts in this report? A related question is, how courageous will the American free press be? Only time will tell.

In February 1937, while still attempting to arrange Dr. Gruner's transfer to San Diego, Johnson wrote to Canada's most esteemed cancer researcher, Dr. Edward Archibald. In the course of the lengthy letter, Johnson explained the Committee's reasons for not making a public announcement at that time. Archibald had earlier asked Johnson about the Committee's silence and also passed on the concerns of McGill's Dr. Martin about the same failure to announce. Johnson replied:

> "We realize that while there has been a distinctly apparent change in the attitude of the medical profession toward the etiology of cancer during the last few years, any announcement we make will be met with tremendous scepticism, and we must make assurance doubly sure before we publish.
>
> "We hope that you will not feel that we are asking too much in urging that Dr. Gruner come to the Rife Laboratory and collaborate with us in the final report. If you and Dr. Gruner agree to this, perhaps we can give the world a real contribution on the etiology of cancer before the end of 1937.
>
> "Our Committee has decided that the etiology of cancer must first be established before we publish anything concerning the possible treatment. We are, therefore, going to let the Rife Ray rest until this most important work is done."

So that was it. A committee chose to be silent about a treatment which already had cured cancer. The cautious doctors preferred to carefully develop the etiology of cancer to the point where it was incontestable. People would die while the group mind of the committee played it super safe. It was a senseless and probably immoral decision, especially when they failed to get Dr. Gruner anyway, thus losing any immediate chance to prove the etiology in a way that could not be challenged. It would have been better to go ahead and make the announcement about the treatment, bring in the existing skeptics and let them see the clinical, day-by-day miracles. But they didn't do it.

Funny, how men often think they have forever. It is a fault which is passed down from generation to generation. Even today there are those making the same mistake. They want to test the Rife treatment again and again, and they say that after a year or so of careful scientific work which will be "incontestable," an announcement will be made. Shakespeare could write a modern tragedy about such men's folly.

On March 31, 1937, C. I. Martin, Faculty of Medicine, Office of the Dean, McGill University, Montreal, informed

Johnson that "you will not be able to get him (Gruner) for the present." Martin then wrote that he and his wife were leaving on a vacation to Italy. The cure for cancer could wait.

Unfortunately, Gruner never was able to go to San Diego. Rife continued a correspondence with him, and Johnson later sent Gruner his own Frequency Instrument—one of the finest then in existence. But this was after the AMA had closed down most of the treatments. Gruner became too frightened to use it. He gave the Frequency Instrument to a priest who was a ham operator, and one of the greatest technologies of the 20th century ended up being used as spare parts for a short-wave radio!

Meanwhile, the difficulties were mounting. Rife had to visit Louisville, Kentucky again in May 1937 because of continued problems with his eyes. In April, Dr. Walker of the Hooper Foundation had to quit the work because of illness. Another doctor was assigned, but he accomplished nothing. The San Francisco research was essentially finished by mid-1937. Johnson reported that the San Francisco surgeons had proved totally uncooperative. In the year and a half that Walker worked, he was able to get only "5 or 6 tumors" from his surgical colleagues.

On May 28, 1937, Dr. Milbank Johnson closed the third clinic. On June 1, he wrote to his friend Dr. Joseph D. Heitger in Louisville, Kentucky, the eye specialist to whom he had sent Rife:

"I closed my clinic on May 28, having been running it for eight months. Our special effort this past winter has been working on cataracts, and while we have treated a number of other infectious conditions (if cataract is an infection), still our principal work has been on the eye.

"The application of the Rife Ray as we have used it, does, in the great majority of cases, restore the full visual function of the eye; that is, the portion of visual disturbance due to opacities in the lens. How it does it and why it does it, I do not know, but the above statement is an actual fact, supported now by many cases.

"How I wish we could get together and go over this work. I believe it will result in epochal changes in the profession's handling of cataract cases."

84

Johnson spent the summer of 1937 in La Jolla outside San Diego. There he worked with Dr. Couche who continued to use the Frequency Instrument in treatment.

In the fall of 1937, Phil Hoyland, the engineer whom Johnson had introduced to Rife, moved to San Diego to begin with three others the commercial manufacturing of the Frequency Instrument. The company was named "Beam Ray." It would play a crucial part in the AMA's destruction of Rife's cancer cure. Hoyland would become the agent of the AMA and would sue Beam Ray with an expensive Los Angeles attorney representing him while the AMA pressured the doctors behind-the-scenes to stop using the Frequency Instruments or lose their license to practice medicine.

The trial would start Rife on a long road of deterioration, alcoholism and depression . . . as the deaths from cancer mounted year after year.

Johnson's introduction of Philip Hoyland into the Rife research and treatment program was undoubtedly one of his most serious miscalculations. Hoyland was a capable electrical engineer and Johnson saw the talent . . . but not the man's character. This error of Johnson's may have contributed to his own suspicious death in 1944 and the end of the Special Research Committee which came so close to telling the world that a cure for cancer and other infectious diseases had been found.

But that disaster was still in the years ahead. Johnson returned to Los Angeles in the fall of 1937 and began treating patients again with the Frequency Instrument. Despite the obstacles and setbacks of 1937, progress continued with the development of the machines. Scientists in various locations were interested. The future seemed hopeful. But any optimism was a mirage. A storm was building and soon would break over San Diego.

Chapter 13
1938: Beam Ray

Beam Ray began in 1937 after Philip Hoyland moved to San Diego from Los Angeles. He was an electrical engineer, had worked with Rife, and had contributed to the improvement of the Frequency Instrument. Rife brought him to the Rife Laboratory in Point Loma on Alcott Street, San Diego.

Hoyland met a promoter named Hutcheson who originated the idea of commercially manufacturing the Frequency Instrument. James Couche, the San Diego doctor who had been treating patients with the Frequency Instrument for some time, was another partner in Beam Ray, along with Ben Cullen, Rife's old friend from the time he arrived in San Diego in 1913.

They approached Rife with the idea and he considered it for some time. Then he gave his approval on two conditions:

"1. That they would adhere decidedly to the original basic principles of the Frequency Instrument.

2. That each Frequency Instrument would be thoroughly tested before delivery to determine its true devitalizing power and effect on pathogenic bacteria."

Fourteen Frequency Instruments were built by Beam Ray. Two went to England, a third to Dr. Hamer, and a fourth to Dr. Arthur Yale. Two more went to Arizona doctors and the remaining eight went to Southern California doctors.

In May 1938, Dr. B. Winter Gonin, W. V. Blewett, and an associate named Parsons arrived from England. They agreed to purchase a microscope from Rife and they discussed selling the microscopes to the world from London. They also met the Beam Ray people and purchased the first two Frequency Instruments (prior to their manufacture).

However, when the two instruments were sent in July and August, they were unwired. Hoyland apparently was seeking a trip to England. The three Englishmen were outraged. Rife had been out of San Diego when the machines were sent. Thus, they had not been tested by him as Beam Ray had agreed.

After an exchange of letters with the Englishmen, Rife agreed to send his assistant Henry Siner to England at the end of the year. Siner would bring a microscope and help the Englishmen establish a laboratory. Rife would follow in mid-1939 and bring the microscope the Englishmen had ordered.

Meanwhile, Dr. Couche had cured a man that most of the San Diego doctors had failed to help. Word of the instrument's healing power was spreading. Dr. Richard Hamer of the Paradise Valley Sanitarium rented the third Beam Ray Frequency Instrument and installed it in the Sanitarium. However, as soon as the other doctors began losing patients, Hamer was forced to remove the Frequency Instrument. So he and an assistant opened an office in National City.

Ben Cullen, the President of Beam Ray, later recalled what happened once Dr. Hamer had his own office:

"Hamer ran an average of forty cases a day through his place. He had to hire two operators. He trained them and watched them very closely . . . Hamer was very well known on the Pacific Coast. His case histories were absolutely wonderful.

"We would go in there and see rectal cancers and stuff of that sort. He cleaned them up completely, absolutely clean. People would come in there with syphilis—not for that purpose—but those that had developed cancers, he'd find they had syphilis or gonorrhea. By golly he'd clean those up completely. Not a doggone taint of it in the blood stream at all. Clinically cured.

"I would go down to Dr. Hamer and he would painstakingly pull out those case histories showing improvement day by day of every one of them."

It was the treatment of the 82 year old man from Chicago by Dr. Hamer that resulted in Morris Fishbein, the AMA head in Chicago, learning about the Frequency Instrument. He then tried to "buy in" through representatives of his from Los

Angeles. When the offer was refused, expensive legal assistance from Los Angeles suddenly was made available to Philip Hoyland.

Hoyland felt he wasn't getting his fair share. Having worked with Rife in building the instruments, he began seeing Cullen, Dr. Couche and the promoter Hutcheson as less important than he. Cullen had used his money to form the corporation. Each member had received 6,000 shares. But Hoyland had the information on the frequencies and tried to use it to gain more shares. Dissatisfied and in disagreement with his partners, he joined forces with the AMA to destroy or take over Beam Ray. His law suit was a naked maneuver to gain control of Beam Ray. By owning Beam Ray, he'd have been in a position to negotiate with Fishbein or any other outsider trying to "buy in."

The trial in 1939 destroyed Rife, led to the disintegration of Beam Ray, stopped the Special Research Committee's carefully developed program and ended most of the clinical work which was healing cancer and other diseases.

Chapter 14
1939: The Storm Breaks

While Rife and his associates were creating a science of the future, they were living in a scientific world of the past—vastly different from the one in which the medical research goliaths were taking shape and which would dominate postwar society. These were vast enterprises linked to powerful financial interests. A breakthrough of the kind Rife was engineering would threaten not only massive investments but even the political empires behind them. Thus, it was not only the doctors but leading scientific authorities of the "monomorphism church" who were ready to oppose Rife and those whose research supported his discoveries. Two examples provide a valuable historic picture of the difference between Rife's smaller world and that which he unknowingly was challenging—a world linking the doctor's union, the health megacities, and the huge financial investments behind them—as well as the government's politicized involvement in medical research.

Henry Siner, Rife's assistant, passed through New York in January 1939 on his way to England where he would demonstrate the microscope and assist in the establishment of a Rife-like English laboratory. While in New York, he visited a Dr. Carscarden and was shown "the medical center." Siner was awe-struck, but he also opened the eyes of those still in the stone age of bacteriology. A letter of Siner's to Rife:

"I just returned from the medical center after having seen Dr. Carscarden and delivered to him the filter, and also instructed him as to its capabilities and use. Dr. Carscarden is one of the finest men I have ever met and I am sure that you and he would get along famously as his line of thought runs so much similar to yours. Since Dr. Carscarden is a surgeon he made me acquainted with the department of research bacteriology and I had a very interesting discussion with those who are trying to unveil the mystery of filter-passing, pathogenic micro-organisms.

"At this point I was impressed with a very unusual and inconsistent spectacle. At least 10 tremendous buildings that have their upper extremities somewhere in the clouds make up the series of institutions known as the medical center. I was awe-struck by the gigantic proportions of the structures, the nurses, patients, and what not that milled and pushed through the halls—Great God—what a mad-house . . . and on the fifth floor, in a little room, out of the way, I beheld the department of bacteriology (research). I swear, Dr. Rife, that the whole laboratory would fit nicely in our dark room, and still leave sufficient space in which to do our developing. It brought to my mind what you have said many times about how badly the important work is neglected.

"The people at work in the lab were engaged in the process of inoculating something into fertile chicken eggs, but were good enough to take the time to explain that they were working on the virus of the cold and the 'flu.' Dr. Carscarden, at this point, announced that I was taking a microscope to England that would reveal these virus forms. He was promptly informed by one of the chief technicians that such a thing was a myth, or words to that effect.

"In the meantime I noticed a copy of Kendall's *Bacteriology* lying on the desk. I picked it up and asked if those assembled thought the author of that book knew anything about the subject, and in the same breath, spread out a reprint of Kendall's (and your) article in the California and Western Medicine, and also a copy of Rosenow's publication in the Mayo Bulletin.

"After this was read aloud by one of the group, the atmosphere was changed quite a little and I noticed that they all stopped working to see what else I had to say—which was plenty. When I got through, any one of them were ready to give a right eye or at least a left eye to see the microscope. I explained that it was impossible at present, but perhaps upon our return from England it might be arranged."

Later that same year, Dr. Gruner of Canada wrote to Milbank Johnson, explaining his frustrations and the reality of the scientific orthodoxy dominating Canada, the Rockefeller Institute in New York, and the Washington research laboratories:

"The crux of the whole problem is the identification of the 'virus,' otherwise 'BX' not only in itself, but also when admixed with other matter. BX now goes by the name of 'elementary bodies.' The center of controversy is now in the question of just what those bodies are. I myself consider them to be the same as BX. Well, the subject came up some time ago when Dr. Archibald and myself called upon Rous at the Rockefeller to see the work on the Shope virus and the term 'elementary bodies' came up, when I showed my photographs of 'my' e-b. He seemed much surprised that I should have found any."

(Note: Rous found the first cancer-causing "virus" in 1911 but wasn't awarded the Nobel Prize until 1966 when he was 86 years old.)

"After that, the subject of the Glover organism came up, and we went to Washington to see the work there on that organism. . . . After long drawn-out consideration I decided for my part that Glover's ultramicroscopic phase was the same as BX and 'e-b', but of course the question (whether this ultramicroscopic phase can develop into cocci and then bacilli) was a very different one. . . . The Department of Public Health at Washington had undergone change of management . . . as they *had just about decided to close down* the Glover work as useless.

"About the same time, but earlier by about three weeks, an immunologist was appointed here by Dr. Archibald, and a bacteriologist as well, both trained and approved by the Prof. of Bacteriology, to check up my work, with a strong bias against the existence of any cancer germ at all. From that time to this, a period of nearly nine months, progress has virtually ceased.

"It was a loss that I could not 'get' your careful expositions of that subject in relation to the action of BX. Since that memorable occasion of being in your company, so much has flown on in regard to the 'phages,' and yet so little is the subject a topic of study in the Universities (I think). However, the conception of 'mutation,' 'pleomorphism,' 'developmental cycles of bacteria' has been uppermost in our thoughts (Dr. Archibald and myself). The battle is between the 'monomorphists' and the 'pleomorphists.' To me, bacteriology is an effete product or dead thing under the current academic view, whereas the other concept not only explains so much that we see in nature, but is actually demonstrated in the microphoto-graphs in the textbooks themselves. It is clear that the authors have never unraveled their own photographs, or else they would see that cocci become bacilli all the time!

"Dr. Rife has, of course, the indispensable tool to effect the proofs. To this day the opticians say that what he did cannot be done. The people in London, whom I interviewed last year about it, were very scornful, and brought out the age-old argu-ment about wave-lengths (I think Dr. Archibald quietly is amused at them, too; it is so like the Galileo busi-ness) . . . The BX may not be 'ultramicroscopic,' it is just not seen because the light used does not show it up, as Dr. Rife demonstrated in his laboratory that time.

"All this goes to show that I myself support Rife's findings as much as ever. I still think his instrument is of supreme value. But even if it were available in many more places, few there are who will trouble to scrutinise the things they work with. We established that with few exceptions the people who work with viruses never look at their material microscopically; they never look at their tumors except with routine haematox-ylin sections; they certainly never examine the living tissues. Even the wonderful cinematograph pictures of the Lewises contain the particles we consider etiological, and they never notice these objects at all—dancing about all over the place, much like BX—but the dance does not interest them!"

This inability to "see" what is right in front of them is one of the reasons cancer researchers have failed to find the cause of cancer (the other reason is the politics involved). In 1983, the Nobel Prize was awarded to Barbara McClintock for her work in gene research. A biography of McClintock by Evelyn Fox Keller titled *A Feeling For the Organism* describes how McClintock learned to *see* in a special way. It is essentially what Gruner was writing about in 1939. He not only had seen Rife's work validated but witnessed a myriad of researchers who could have seen something similar without Rife's aid—if they had looked. Keller describes how Nobel Prize winner McClintock and other first class scientists looked and "saw" in a special way:

"For all of us, our concepts of the world build on what we see, as what we see builds on what we think. Where we know more, we see more. . . .

94

"What is it in an individual scientist's relation to nature that facilitates the kind of seeing that eventually leads to productive discourse? What enabled McClintock to see further and deeper into the mysteries of genetics than her colleagues?

"Her answer is simple. Over and over again, she tells us one must have the time to look, the patience to 'hear what the material has to say to you,' the openness to 'let it come to you.' Above all, one must have a 'feeling for the organism.'

"This intimate knowledge, made possible by years of close association with the organism she studies, is a prerequisite for her extraordinary perspicacity. 'I have learned so much about the corn plant that when I see things, I can interpret (them) right away.' Both literally and figuratively, her 'feeling for the organism' has extended her vision."

Rife sitting in his chair with the microscope for as long as 48 hours without moving demonstrates the extent to which he was devoted to this process of "seeing." And compared to the army of microbiologists who couldn't see even the obvious (as Gruner noted) these opponents of Rife—defending their turf and using their powerful positions at the Rockefeller Institute and Harvard to attack Kendall or Rife—now can be recognized for what they were: inferior scientists.

Rosenow's son told this writer that his father eventually became philosophical about such inferior scientists as Rivers and Zinsser. Rosenow Sr. said to his son, "Edward, no matter how hard I try to convince others, nothing happens unless an occasional person opens his mind and is willing to listen" (or in the case of Rife, opens his eyes in order to see).

This little preamble prepares the stage for the trial of 1939. It was really two men facing off—one was a scientist who could see (Rife), the other was a political power addict whose scientific credentials were mediocre at best and whose commercial ethics were, to say the least, suspect (Fishbein).

Morris Fishbein graduated from Rush Medical School. He interned for only six months and never practiced medicine a day in his life. His mentor, a man named Simpson, also was a product of Rush Medical School. Simpson, as head of the AMA Journal, had developed the lucrative structure which enabled the AMA to be dominated by dictatorial whims. In 1922, Simpson was forced to resign after a court case in which it was shown he had falsely tried to have his wife committed to an insane asylum. She showed in court that Simpson had made her a drug addict. Such was the background of the early AMA founders—essentially second-rate doctors in their own time who used the organization to gain power and make money. The public welfare was a secondary consideration. The New York Times obituary for Fishbein in the 1970s reported that he had entered medicine because as a young man he had perceived the "power" which a doctor had. Power was his driving personal motive, not healing. His autobiography is little more than an egotistic memoir of all the famous people he met in his life.

Yet Fishbein controlled the AMA and also intimidated the press and other institutions to such an extent that his actions, no matter how heinous, could go virtually unchallenged. Unfortunately, the situation has not changed very much today. When a group of cancer patients from around the country protested the inaccuracies in a *Journal of the AMA* article about a cancer clinic in the Bahamas, a number of media people apologized to the patient's group because the media could not print the true facts. (This is 1985!) The reason? "The rebuttal would cut them off from their primary source and render them impotent journalists." The head of the patient's group, Jack Link of Kalamazoo, Michigan concluded that the journalists "are already impotent."

Such was the organization Rife faced during the 1939 trial— a powerful medical union which played by its own rules, ignored the law, promoted products which were unhealthy, intimidated the press, politicians and medical researchers, and unfortunately perverted basic principles of the American nation.

Rife was about to leave for England in May 1939 when he was subpoenaed. The trial opened on June 12, 1939 with Judge Edward Kelly presiding. On one side was Philip Hoyland backed by his high-priced legal talent. Alone against them stood local San Diego attorney Bert Comperet. The opposing lawyer tore into Rife in a way he had never experienced. His nerves gave. A doctor recommended that he take a drink to calm himself. Rife's alcoholism began.

Ben Cullen's remembrance of this period includes the following:

> "Well Rife was called in to testify two or three times. Judge Kelly was a wonderful man, but Rife had never been in court and he just became a nervous jibbering idiot, in that he couldn't stand it and he did his best to keep calm, his hands shaking like a leaf of course. He had started smoking pretty heavily and inhaling it which he didn't use to do before. Anyway he took to drinking because the doctor couldn't find anything to stop his nervousness without forcing him into a drug addict. Finally he got so he had to crave it.
>
> "Afterwards, during his clear moments when he wasn't under the influence of liquor, he would endeavor to progress but every doggone day at a certain time he would go and get one little nip out of his car and that was the end of it."

While the court case was taking place (and afterwards), the AMA visited all the doctors involved. Those who didn't stop using the Frequency Instrument would lose their medical license. Dr. Hamer quickly returned his instrument. Other kinds of pressure were put on the Special Research Committee members. Milbank Johnson apparently didn't budge. He sent his own Frequency Instrument to Dr. Gruner in 1942, still hoping for the international confirmation which would enable him to proclaim the cure for cancer in a way that was incontestable. But Gruner was to disappoint him by not using it out of fear. Johnson's *Who's Who* biographical information for 1944 emphasized that "now" (in 1944) he was still head of the committee, still fighting for a way to bring Rife's discoveries to the world. But most of the others beat hasty retreats.

After Johnson's death in 1944, the records of the committee were destroyed. Cullen remembered:

> "It was so controversial. They (the University of Southern California) were scared to death."

Mystery shrouds Johnson's death. One rumor is that he was preparing to announce the cure for cancer just before he was hospitalized. The suspicion exists that he was silenced, but the evidence is circumstantial. However, two federal inspectors did examine his hospital record in the late 1950s-early 1960s. They concluded it was likely that he was poisoned.

Sometime in the 1944-46 period, a new technician in Rife's laboratory stole one of the valuable quartz prisms from the Universal Microscope, rendering it inoperable. Just prior to the theft, Dr. Raymond Seidel had published a description of the microscope in the Smithsonian annual report. The report described how the cancer virus "may be observed to succumb when exposed to certain lethal frequencies." This was the news which the opponents of Rife were determined to have suppressed. Publication in the Smithsonian report was a dangerous breach of their wall of censorship. Following the publication, Seidel soon became aware that he was being followed. Then a bullet crashed through his car windshield while he was driving.

Dr. Couche continued using the Frequency Instrument (until the mid-1950s). He defied the AMA and had his membership revoked.

Dr. Royal Lee of the Lee Foundation for Nutritional Research in Milwaukee, Wisconsin spent many weekends with Royal Rife. He later published a small report on the Fishbein-Rife tragedy. It includes the following:

> "No medical journal was ever permitted to report on Rife's work. This one by the Franklin Institute slipped by the censors, since this organization is not medical but supports general scientific activities. But that mistake was soon rectified, it appears, as there is still no general knowledge of Rife's epoch-making discoveries. Again, the iron curtain of Fishbein is effective. . . . We can give a list of various subjects on which this censorship is rigorously applied. Only the treatment of disease with synthetic drugs is carefully reported. Botanicals are played down, foods as remedies are almost as taboo as Rife's work . . . the official definition of a medical remedy for disease . . . excludes automatically any vitamin, nutritional mineral or enzyme . . ."

Beam Ray won the case against Philip Hoyland. Judge Kelly stated at the end of the trial, "The court is not called upon to pass on the merits of this machine. But the people here before the court have great confidence in its powers, both curative and money making." As for Hoyland, Kelly had judged his character accurately. Kelly: "I am not convinced of his blameless chracter in these transactions as to find that he is in court with that degree of manly cleanliness that the court insists upon. He stands alone and opposed to the directors of the corporation. The court has confidence in their honesty and integrity. . . . I am denying the plaintiff (Hoyland) has clean hands. I am denying him the relief he demands because I don't believe he was above trying to get an advantage for himself in every transaction. . . . I am holding that the man who asked relief here is not in equity with clean hands, and I say again I'll not give him relief."

While the AMA's role behind-the-scene did not come up in court, Judge Kelly must have learned about it. When the trial was over, Kelly offered to represent Beam Ray in a new suit against the AMA. But Ben Cullen was broke. He had even lost his house. He got a job and left the cure for cancer to others. Rife kept his laboratory intact until 1946, but his drinking eventually forced him to sell it piece by piece.

So, although the AMA lost its court case against Beam Ray, it won the war. But millions of Americans suffering from cancer decade after decade would lose. Fishbein's action in 1939 makes him, in this writer's opinion, the worst mass murderer in American history.

Note: Just prior to the attack on Rife in the spring of 1939, the only other quality "electronic medicine research lab" in America was mysteriously destroyed by fire. For 15 years, J. C. Burnett's lab in New Jersey had conducted research and kept records on "electronic energy in its relationship to the human body." The $250,000 lab (1924 dollars) on a 400 acre estate, and more than $500,000 invested in research, were financed by Burnett's wife, the former Cora B. Timken of the Timken Roller Bearing family. It was her relative on the west coast who had first financed Rife. The lab was burned to the ground while Burnett and his wife were visiting Rife in California—a strange coincidence in that dark, pivotal year of 1939!

Chapter 15

The Microscope and the
Frequency Instrument

From the perspective of the mid-1980s, the greatest mistake in the long ordeal of the 1930s probably happened on May 3-4, 1932 when Kendall addressed the Association of American Physicians in Baltimore. Sitting in the audience waiting to pounce were Dr. Rivers and Dr. Zinsser. Neither had been able to reproduce the effects which Kendall showed were possible using his "K Medium". But potential allies also were in that audience such as the great William Welch.

Kendall had a right to be proud of his achievement, but it was a catastrophic error in judgment for him to ignore the Rife microscope in his talk and especially in his defense after Rivers and Zinsser had essentially called him a liar. Kendall had already published with Rife a description of their combined achievement. All he had to do was simply state that a great new microscope made the filter-passing forms visible to the eye. Without access to the microscope, Rivers and Zinsser had no argument.

But Kendall did not mention Rife. If he had, all the researchers who would later read the description of the meeting (in the Journal of the AMA for the summer of 1932) would have focused on the microscope instead of the monomorphism versus pleomorphism feud. Publishing the discovery in the Journal of the AMA in 1932—long before Rife became a threat to the AMA—might have changed the history of later years. If nothing else the microscope's abilities would have been more widely known and Rife's authority would have been harder to attack seven years later when it was his cancer curing instruments which were the subject of litigation.

But Kendall tried to gain too much glory for himself. He

became the object of brutal attack when he had at his disposal a weapon which could have quickly silenced his opponents' offensive.

Kendall himself later came under the heavier guns which were employed in the 1940s to wipe out the memory of the cancer cure. He was an authority whose "K Medium" was crucial to Rife's discoveries. Ben Cullen's memories include this sad conclusion to Kendall's brilliant career:

> "I think Kendall was paid off about $200,000. He went down deep into Mexico and he bought a ranch to that tune, and the Mexicans cleaned him out of that. So he is living off his son-in-law in La Jolla." (1958)

Kendall died the following year in the town where the 1934 clinic had cured cancer. There was something odd—even mystical—about the way in which people associated with the cancer cure found their way to La Jolla, as will be seen when the later story of Dr. Virginia Livingston-Wheeler is summarized.

But even with Kendall's silence in Baltimore, the opportunity for American microbiologists to put aside the silly monomorphism versus pleomorphism debate and focus on what the microscope showed, was still there. Yet few chose to do so.

Rosenow's two reports in the summer of 1932—one in the Mayo Clinic's publication and the other in *Science* magazine—clearly provided the crucial facts to the scientific community. From Rosenow's *Science* article of August 26, 1932:

> "Examination under the Rife microscope of specimens, containing objects visible with the ordinary microscope, leaves no doubt of the accurate visualization of objects or particulate matter by direct observation at the extremely high magnification (calculated to 8,000 diameters) obtained with this instrument."

Other scientists simply wouldn't look. As Dr. Gruner's 1939 letter made clear, the microscope authorities did not want to believe such a microscope existed. The old "light frequency" argument came up and still can be heard when microscopists and physicists are told about the Rife microscope in the mid-1980s. Rife's microscope contradicted the most cherished beliefs of the experts—then and now.

When the electron microscope began to be introduced in 1940-41, Rife made a trip to Germany. He recognized immediately that it was inferior to what he had built in 1929. His microscope could see living organisms. The electron microscope killed its specimens. As one expert in 1986 noted in discussing this "live" micro-organism versus "dead" micro-organism matter, the existing authorities will have to learn to "see" all over again. A generation of scientists have grown up on the electron microscope. The world of living micro-organisms is totally alien to them.

It need not have been if Rife's microscope and Rife's Frequency Instrument weren't suppressed by ignorant men in control of power and resources beyond any kind of public accountability. One can only imagine what could have evolved from Rife's two great discoveries if a generation of scientists had been allowed to develop and improve them while gaining new knowledge of deadly micro-organisms and how their painless destruction extended human well-being.

In 1938, Rife made his most public announcement. In a two part article written by Newall Jones of the San Diego *Evening Tribune* (May 6 and May 11), Rife said, "We do not wish at this time to claim that we have 'cured' cancer, or any other disease, for that matter. But we can say that these waves, or this ray, as the frequencies might be called, have been shown to possess the power of devitalizing disease organisms, of 'killing' them, when tuned to an exact wave length, or frequency, for each different organism. This applies to the organisms both in their free state and, with certain exceptions, when they are in living tissues."

In 1953, Rife was not so conservative. In his copyrighted explanation of his work and discoveries, he states 14 of 16 cases of cancer and other diseases were cured in 1934 when the BX cancer frequency was turned on them for three minutes every third day. (The other two were pronounced cured one month after the clinic closed.)

In 1942, four years after the San Diego news report, Dr. Raymond E. Seidel began investigating the microscope for an article. At one point, he spent 3 weeks in Rife's Laboratory. In February 1944, the article appeared in the Journal of the Franklin Institute. It was reprinted later that year in the Annual Report of the Smithsonian Institution. Because Seidel was a medical doctor and not a microscope expert, his description was not in the technical terminology to which narrow-minded microscope authorities were accustomed. Microscope experts in the 1980s have sneered at his lack of technical vocabulary. Nevertheless, more open-minded experts then and now were excited by his report. Letters from laboratories came to Rife as much as 4 years after the publication, pleading for information. Unfortunately, by then Rife's laboratory was closed and Rife was slowly selling it off piece-by-piece in order to eat. Dr. Seidel mentioned the 5,682 parts of the Universal Microscope and then described how it differed from ordinary microscopes:

"Between the source of light and the specimen are subtended two circular, wedge-shaped, block crystal quartz prisms for the purpose of polarizing the light passing through the specimen, polarization being the practical application of the theory that light waves vibrate in all planes perpendicular to the direction in which they are propagated. Therefore, when light comes into contact with a polarizing prism, it is divided or split into two beams, one of which is refracted to such an extent that it is reflected to the side of the prism without, of course, passing through the prism while the second ray, bent considerably less, is thus enabled to pass through the prism to illuminate the specimen. . . . Now, when the portion of the spectrum is reached in which both the organism and the color band vibrate in exact accord, one with the other, a definite characteristic spectrum is emitted by the organism. . . .

"Now, instead of the light rays starting up the tube in a parallel fashion, tending to converge as they rise higher and finally crossing each other, arriving at the ocular separated by considerable distance as would be the case with an ordinary microscope, in the universal tube the rays also start their rise parallel to each other but, just as they are about to cross, a specially designed quartz prism is inserted which serves to pull them out parallel again, another prism being inserted each time the rays are about to cross. . . . Thus, the greatest distance that the image in the universal is projected through any one media, either quartz or air, is 30 millimeters instead of the 160, 180, or 190 millimeters as in the empty or air-filled tube of an ordinary microscope. . . .

"Under the universal microscope disease organisms such as those of tuberculosis, cancer, sarcoma, streptococcus, typhoid, staphylococcus, leprosy, hoof and mouth disease, and others may be observed to succumb when exposed to certain lethal frequencies peculiar to each individual organism, and directed upon them by rays covering a wide range of waves. By means of a camera attachment and a motion-picture camera not built into the instrument, many 'still' micrographs as well as hundreds of feet of motion-picture film bear witness to the complete life cycles of numerous organisms. It should be emphasized, perhaps, that invariably the same organisms refract the same colors when stained by means of the mono-chromatic beam of illumination on the universal microscope, regardless of the media upon which they are grown. The virus of the *Bacillus typhosus* is always a turquoise blue, the *Bacillus coli* always mahogany colored, the *Mycobacterium leprae* always a ruby shade, the filter-passing form or virus of tuberculosis is always an emerald green, the virus of cancer always a purplish red, and so on."

Rife's copyrighted explanation of 1953 describes the Universal Microscope's unique design as follows:

"The prime reason that viruses have never been observed in their true form of their association with a disease is because the best standard research microscopes will not show them; first, on account of the lack of great enough magnification and second, owing to the minuteness of these particles, it is impossible to stain them with any known method or technique using acid or aniline dye stains hence a substitute stain was found. The viruses were stained with a frequency of light that coordinates with the chemical constituents of the particle or micro-organism under observation.

"The variation of the light frequency is accomplished by use of a variable monochromatic beam of light that is tuned to coordinate with the chemical constituents of particle, virus, or micro-organism. Visibility of the particle, virus, or micro-organism is observed by use of the core beams from the patented Rife Microscope Lamps, which provide illumination through a series of rotating quartz prisms in the universal microscope and thence through the slide containing the specimens and on to the eyepiece. Rotation of the light beams in the quartz prisms controls the increase or decrease of the light frequency. With complete control of the illuminating unit, a frequency is created that is in coordination with the chemical constituents of the virus under observation and thus it is possible to observe the virus in its true chemical refractive index. The control of the illumination (in the universal microscope) is a most important factor in visualizing the virus of any pathogenic micro-organism. This cannot be accomplished by any conventional source of illumination. This points out why other research groups have failed to find cancer virus."

The Frequency Instruments were steadily improved from the early version of 1920 to the clinical versions of 1934-38 and then, in the 1950s, improved again to the point where Rife could assert, "they are infallible and simple to operate."

The May 6, 1928 Evening Tribune of San Diego described what the Frequency Instrument did:

"Just what this Ray does to the organisms to devitalize them is not yet known. Because each organism requires a different wave length, it may be that whatever befalls these tiny slayers of man is something similar to the phenomenon occurring when the musical tuning fork is set in vibration by sound waves emanating from another fork struck nearby. . . .

"Rife thinks that the lethal frequencies for various disease organisms are, as in the sound waves, coordinates of frequencies existing in the organism themselves. If this is the explanation, it means that the Rife Ray probably causes the disease organisms to disintegrate or partially disintegrate, just as the vase and the glass. Several bits of evidence indicate that this is exactly what happens. . . .

"When the ray is directed upon them, they are seen to behave very curiously; some kinds do literally disintegrate, and others writhe as if in agony and finally gather together in deathly unmoving clusters.

"Brief exposure to the tuned frequencies, Rife commented, brings the fatal reactions. In some organisms, it happens in seconds.

"After the organisms have been bombarded, the laboratory reports show, they are dead. They have become devitalized— no longer exhibit life, do not propagate their kind and produce no disease when introduced into the bodies of experimental animals.

"Now, he reported, the mortal oscillatory rates for many, many organisms have been found and recorded and the ray can be tuned to a germ's recorded frequency and turned upon that organism with the assurance that the organism will be killed."

In 1950, after an absence of four years, including two years in an alcohol rehabilitation "prison" from which he finally escaped, Rife returned to his great work. In 1953, his cancer report was published—*History of the Development of a Successful Treatment for Cancer and Other Virus, Bacteria and Fungi.*

Three years later, in 1956, he wrote a letter describing the safety of the Frequency Instrument and also its advanced development:

"I have operated the 'Frequency Instrument' since 1921. I have watched it advance in style and performance with the advancement of electronics.

"In the many years I used this equipment in my research, I have never suffered an injury or any ill effects whatsoever. I found it reliable in performance and efficient in results. The most recent model is infallible and simple to operate."

Chapter 16
1946-1986: Rife's Theory Gains Acceptance

Rife was never published or mentioned in any scientific report after the mid-1940s. Those who knew what he had done also knew what had been done *to* him. Even much later, those whose own work confirmed Rife's discoveries and who personally knew Rife avoided mentioning his name. Scientists frequently talk about a "courageous search for truth," but in practice they more often exhibit a cautious silence when their own career and credibility are on the line. Rife was the invisible man of cancer research right up to his death in 1971. Yet his Frequency Instrument continues to be used secretly by a few brave doctors. And still the occasional heroic physician provides a statement about its miraculous effects.

Nevertheless, the development of Rife's treatment for cancer effectively ended in the late 1930s and early 1940s because the essential cross-referencing of experience by a number of doctors was stopped. The Frequency Instrument was improved and perfected by Rife and his new associates in the 1950s, but the open, clinical, enthusiastic testing of the Rife Ray by a committee of top doctors, scientists and pathologists was never repeated. Political interests disguised as public health protectors prevented any objective evaluation.

Instead, the confirmation of Rife's work came from another direction—bacteria studies and gradual verification of the filter-passing form. The next generation did not have the microscope or the Frequency Instrument, but they proved that the cancer virus exists, that it can change forms, and that it can be destroyed. The approach was through vaccine and diet. It was certainly more complicated (and much more expensive than Rife's easy 3 minute frequency treatment), but the goal was the same—a genuine cure for cancer in place of the failed "approved treatments" of surgery, radiation and chemotherapy.

The key person in the succeeding generation's discovery of the cancer micro-organism was Dr. Virginia Wuerthele-Caspe (Wuerthe was her maiden name and Caspe the name of her first husband). With her second marriage to Dr. Livingston, she changed her name to Dr. Virginia Wuerthele-Caspe-Livingston. After her third marriage, she was known as Dr. Virginia Livingston-Wheeler. To avoid confusion, the name Dr. Virginia Livingston-Wheeler will be used here even if the period cited is prior to her taking that name.

In the summer of 1947, the year following the closing of Rife's laboratory, while living on the East Coast, Dr. Livingston-Wheeler began studying tumors and found the same organism in all of them. In 1948, she came across the work of Dr. Eleanor Alexander-Jackson who, according to Livingston-Wheeler, had demonstrated that the tubercle bacillus went through many changes. (This was the same discovery Kendall, Rosenow and Rife had shown in the early 1930s, but it had been forgotten.)

Dr. Livingston-Wheeler was fascinated by a bacterium that "could be so wildly pleomorphic." She began seeking the same changes in her cancer organism.

In March 1948, at a symposium with Dr. Roy M. Allen, a microscopist, Dr. Livingston-Wheeler announced her findings. In August 1948, the New York Microscopical Society Bulletin published the paper. It included the following:

"In conclusion, it may be stated that a definite mycobacterium is observed in many kinds of tumors. Its presence within the tumor cells as well as within the blood of the patients suffering with the disease can be demonstrated."

By the end of 1948, Dr. Virginia Livingston-Wheeler and Dr. Eleanor Alexander-Jackson had proof that the Rous cancer virus was in actuality a pleomorphic bacterium.

In 1949, following the announcement in New York by two doctors of a virus associated with cancer, Dr. James Couche traveled to Montreal where he visited Dr. Gruner. The *San*

Diego Union of July 31, 1949 reported Gruner's opinion of the latest discovery:

> "Gruner told Dr. Couche he was satisfied that Dr. Rife's large microscope . . . had revealed a virus. He said further that the work he did with Rife at his Point Loma laboratory and follow-up researches at McGill University, had confirmed that tumorous growths positively could be produced by the virus discovered in San Diego.
>
> "Gruner disclosed that he had been working with Dr. J. E. Hett of Windsor, another cancer specialist, who has been studying malignant growths for 50 years and had found that Hett was having remarkable success with a serum he had developed from a virus.
>
> "In San Diego yesterday Dr. Rife admitted the possibility that the cancer virus reported in New York and the virus developed by Dr. Hett are the same virus he isolated in San Diego. . . . Dr. Rife said, . . . 'I discovered that the virus organism gets in the blood of the victim at one stage of the growth.'
>
> "Dr. Couche said . . . that if cancer is a blood disease it is carried to all parts of the body in the blood stream and surgery would be of little use. . . . It will surely be a great honor for that patient San Diego investigator, Dr. Rife, if his virus turns out to be the entity chiefly responsible for causing this dread disease."

By June 1949, Dr. Livingston-Wheeler had become head of the New Rutgers-Presbyterian Laboratory in Newark, New Jersey.

In 1950, Dr. Irene Corey Diller of the Institute for Cancer Research in Philadelphia had isolated fungus agents from cancerous growths in animals. It was Dr. Gruner's fungus from the blood of cancer victims which Rife had taken, transformed to his BX, and then, reversing the process, changed his BX to Gruner's fungus. Diller independently and unknowingly had confirmed a basic area of Rife and Gruner's work.

Also in 1950, Dr. Diller attempted to set up a symposium in New York in order to announce her discovery. It was killed by Dr. Cornelius P. Rhoads, the powerful head of Memorial Sloan-Kettering Cancer Center. Rhoads was determined to prove that cancer could be cured by killing the cancerous cells.

Anything suggesting a micro-organism caused cancer and that the entire body had to be immunized directly threatened his prestige and his entire cancer program, not to mention the pharmaceutical industry which developed thousands of chemotherapy treatments against cancer cells. Until 1955, most of these new drugs were tested at Memorial Sloan-Kettering Cancer Institute.

The same year brought confirmation of Dr. Livingston-Wheeler's cancer microbe's "pleomorphism" by Dr. James Hillman of RCA Labs in Princeton, N. J. Using an electron microscope, he saw the cancer microbe's "filtered" or smaller form.

In December 1950, the *American Journal of Medical Sciences* published Dr. Livingston-Wheeler's article describing how the cancer culture taken from both humans and animals had produced similar disease in experimental animals. Then new cultures were isolated. They matched. The basic principles of bacteriology—known as Koch's postulates—had been fulfilled. Cancer could result from a bacterium! The dismissal of this claim by Rivers and an army of virologists had been shown to be wrong.

Unfortunately, Dr. Livingston-Wheeler's discovery would have little impact. The cancer hierarchy had its own program and America would march to it for the next 35 years while millions suffered and died for nothing because greed, arrogance and ignorance dominated the medical power centers instead of scientific objectivity.

Later Dr. Diller confirmed that Dr. Livingston-Wheeler's microbe converted normal cells to abnormal cells. In 1953, Dr. Diller finally published her fungus discovery, titled "Studies of Fungoid Forms Found in Malignancy."

Also in 1953, Dr. Livingston-Wheeler and her team presented their discoveries at the 6th International Congress of Microbiology in Rome. Among her group was Dr. George Clark who had labored for 8 years in Washington, D.C. on the Glover virus but had not been permitted to publish his results. Dr. Gruner of Montreal had traveled to Washington in the late 1930s to assess the Glover virus and had concluded it was BX. The health bureaucracy in Washington had man-

112

aged to cover up and eventually ignore this research—as their successors have continued to do until today with other pleomorphic micro-organisms.

The Washington Post of September 10, 1953 reported the group's findings:

"Rome Sep 9—An American research group today pictured cancer as an infectious disease, like tuberculosis or syphilis, caused by a tiny organism. . . . Its members said they have obtained an antiserum from bodies of animals infected with the disease and that the antiserum weakens and sometimes destroys the cancer-causing organism. Drs Virginia Wuerthele-Caspe, Eleanor Alexander-Jackson, W. L. Smith and G. A. Clark of the Presbyterian Hospital, Newark, N.J., said their study of cancer induced in white mice and guinea pigs 'has led to the concept that cancer does not consist of a localized tumor alone.' Instead they pictured it as a generalized disease caused by an organism in the human blood stream."

The report received great attention but the New York Academy of Medicine immediately discounted the announcement. *The Washington Post,* which later would unearth and finally break Watergate in one of the best journalistic efforts of the 20th century, in 1953 meekly accepted the orthodox view and walked away from the greatest medical story of the modern age. It was a pattern that seemed to repeat again and again. Those controlling the cancer program of America continued to demonstrate virtual censorship over what the American public could read in the press about cancer.

When the group returned to America, they discovered that Dr. Rhoads of Memorial Sloan-Kettering Cancer Center had managed to stop the funds for the Rutgers-Presbyterian Hospital Laboratory. The Laboratory was closed. Dr. Livingston-Wheeler was out of work and nowhere on the East Coast was there any research organization that would take her in. She had become, like Rife, "invisible." The micro-organism that caused cancer and the hopeful vaccine which would prevent cancer were unwanted. Surgery, radiation and chemotherapy were the "approved" research areas—as they remain in 1987.

So Virginia Livingston-Wheeler moved to Los Angeles where she worked at the Los Angeles County Hospital. She

113

sought a position with the University of Southern California Medical School—as the threads in this tale begin to cross—but was turned down.

Her father, Dr. Wuerthele, however, had retired and moved to San Diego. In 1955, his daughter followed him. Soon after, her husband Dr Caspe died. She was almost 50, a widow and had a daughter to support. She took a job in a San Diego clinic. Within a year she met Dr. Livingston and married him in 1957.

In 1958, she reemerged on the international cancer scene. On July 14, 1958, the 1st International Congress for Microbiology of Cancer and Leukemia opened in Antwerp. Dr. Livingston-Wheeler was a Vice-President and was given the honor of being the first speaker. She also discovered that the pleomorphism theory of cancer was widely accepted in Europe even though ignored in America. A determined effort to find an immunological treatment was also well-advanced in Europe.

In her 1983 book *The Conquest of Cancer,* Dr. Virginia Livingston-Wheeler wrote:

"All these distinguished scientists, back in 1958, had been carrying on significant research in the biological and immunological treatment of cancer for years. It is still only now that the United States orthodoxy is beginning to catch up. Because of the suppressive actions of the American Cancer Society, the American Medical Association and the Food and Drug Administration, our people have not had the advantage of the European research.

"This work has been ignored because certain powerful individuals backed by large monetary grants can become the dictators of research and suppress all work that does not promote their interests or that may present a threat to their prestige."

In 1959, Dr. Clara Fonti of Milan inoculated herself with a *bacterial* culture of cancer. She grew a tumor. It was surgically removed. The human test had shown what all the laboratory transfers from human blood to human cancer tissue to fungus had shown in cultures or in animals.

And in 1959-1960, Dr. Livingston-Wheeler met a neighbor in San Diego—Royal R. Rife. She had come across a country and connected the years to meet the "invisible man" of cancer research. Some strange quirk of destiny had brought her to the place—La Jolla outside San Diego—where the first clinic which successfully treated cancer was held.

Dr. Livingston-Wheeler often visited Rife's new laboratory in 1959-60. She arranged for the Institute for Cancer Research in Philadelphia to provide mice for Rife and his new associates. This was another strange link because of Rife's earlier unsuccessful association with the International Cancer Research Foundation in Philadelphia. Rife's ideas on pleomorphism closely paralleled those held by Dr. Livingston-Wheeler. The only difference was that Dr. Livingston-Wheeler intended to develop a serum while Rife knew the BX would disintegrate under his Rife Ray.

So they went their separate ways—Livingston-Wheeler to present papers before audiences of elite scientists despite the opposition from the cancer power structure, and Rife to watch his associates be harassed by FDA break-ins, court trials, and continuing AMA pronouncements that the cancer clinic of 1934 was "a myth."

In 1962, Dr. Livingston-Wheeler had a heart attack and was essentially inactive until 1965. But in 1965 she co-authored a paper with her old colleague Dr. Eleanor Alexander-Jackson. In 1966, the two of them appeared at the American Cancer Seminar for Science Writers in Arizona. However, the powers behind the scene still didn't like what the two women were saying. When Dr. Alexander-Jackson returned to Columbia University, she found that her work had been terminated.

In May 1966, Rife and his associates tried to interest the Institute for Cancer Research in Philadelphia in the Frequency Instrument. The Institute backed away. Rife was still the "invisible man" with the cure that never happened.

In 1966, Peyton Rous was awarded the Nobel Prize for his virus discovered in 1911. By that time, it was 18 years since Dr. Virginia Livingston-Wheeler and Dr. Eleanor Alexander-Jackson had proven it was a classic filtered form of a bacterium.

Sometime in the 1960s, Dr. Livingston-Wheeler began taking her own cancer vaccine—once a year.

In 1967, Dr. Irene Diller and Dr. Florence Seibert published a report in the *Annals of the New York Academy of Science* that they had isolated bacteria from every tumor they obtained.

In 1968, Dr. Livingston-Wheeler and her second husband Dr. Livingston opened a cancer clinic in San Diego—where the University of Southern California Special Research Committee had conducted the first cancer clinic using the early Frequency Instrument, curing 14 of 16 patients in 70 days, and the other 2 within 90 days.

From 1968 to 1983, over 10,000 cancer patients were treated at the new clinic. Dr. Livingston-Wheeler reported that they had an 80% success rate.

On November 5-8, 1969, the New York Academy of Sciences welcomed Dr. Livingston-Wheeler and Dr. Eleanor Alexander-Jackson, both representing the University of California at San Diego, Dr. Irene Diller from the Institute of Cancer Research in Philadelphia, and Dr. Florence Seibert from the Veterans Administration Research Laboratory in Bay Pines, Florida. Their topic was "Microorganisms Associated With Malignancy."

Diagnosis News reported that the researchers from three separate institutions had "found a highly pleomorphic organism in all types of human and animal tumors, in the blood of advanced cancer patients. . . .

On October 30, 1970, the Academy published their report. It could have been written by Rife, Johnson, Kendall, Rosenow and Gruner. Like echoes from the 1930s, it stated the truth about cancer with certainty. It also defiantly challenged the cancer establishment's orthodox views:

"Microorganisms of various sorts have been observed and isolated from animal and human tumors, including viruses, bacteria, and fungi. There is, however, one specific type of highly pleomorphic microorganism that has been observed and isolated consistently by us from human and animal malignancies of every obtainable variety for the past 20 years. . . . The organism has remained an unclassified mystery, due in part to its remarkable pleomorphism and its stimulation of other microorganisms. Its various phases may resemble viruses, micrococci, diptheroids, bacilli, and fungi."

In 1971, Royal R. Rife died.

On December 23, 1971, President Richard Nixon signed a $1.6 billion law to open the "war on cancer." And everyone lined up for the feast: the greed merchants at the American Cancer Society, the AMA, research scientists at various favored institutes and universities, the health bureaucrats at the National Cancer Institute, and the politicians. By 1985, the National Cancer Institute was spending $1.2 billion yearly . . . and had precious little to show for it.

In 1972, Dr. Livingston-Wheeler published her first book, *Cancer: A New Breakthrough*. In her 1948 presentation before the New York Microscopic Society, she had said, "170,000 deaths" per year were caused by cancer. By 1972, the figures were much worse: "350,000 deaths a year." By 1986, there would be 460,000 deaths every year—all unnecessary. And with the rapid spread of AIDS, a disease which Dr. Livingston-Wheeler and associates of Rife claimed could be cured, the National Academy of Sciences in late 1986 called for $2 billion a year to avert "a national health crisis." 60,000 deaths a year from AIDS were predicted by the 1990s.

Dr. Livingston-Wheeler in her 1972 book condemned the National Cancer Institute for its misuse of money, the corrupt handling of its public health responsibilities, and its use of people as guinea pigs for a "surgery-radiation-chemotherapy" program dictated by special interests. Her denunciation of the past would correctly describe the worsening "cancer war" of the future from 1972 to 1986:

> "In thirteen years the NCI has spent five hundred million dollars and has tested 170,000 poisonous drugs for possible use in the fight against cancer. The results have been zero except in a few rare types of cancer. Over 100,000 cancer patients have been used as guinea pigs without their full knowledge and informed consent."

In 1974, Lida Mattman published *Cell-Wall Deficient Forms,* decisively showing the existence of pleomorphic bacteria and relating its early examination to a "school of filtration" established by Kendall. A disguised hint of recognition for Royal R. Rife finally had appeared in the serious scientific literature.

117

In October of 1974, doctors and scientists from around the world gathered at the New York Academy of Sciences to discuss "the interaction of electricity and living systems." One doctor predicted that, by 1994, "electrotherapy" would be used as much as chemotherapy. He bemoaned the fact that current medical students, who would be doctors for the next 40 years, were not being instructed in electrical engineering. Not one of the eminent professionals in "electronic medicine" was aware of Rife's clinical results 30 years earlier.

In 1975, Dr. Livingston died and Dr. Livingston-Wheeler was a widow for the second time.

In 1976, two strange events occurred which seemed to draw together the closing ends of a great circle. Christopher Bird authored the first article to appear on Rife since the 1940s. "What Has Become of the Rife Microscope?" appeared in *New Age Journal* for March 1976. And that same year, Dr. Virginia Livingston-Wheeler married Dr. Owen Wheeler, one of the founders of Doctors Hospital in San Diego. The Livingston Clinic became the Livingston-Wheeler Clinic. A circle of 42 years was complete because Dr. Wheeler, as a young man, had known Royal R. Rife and had been at his side in the Rife Laboratory.

In 1980, the two French scientists Sorin Sonea and Maurice Panisset published *A New Bacteriology*. Bacterial pleomorphism was the key to this "new" bacteriology.

In 1984, Dr. Virginia Livingston-Wheeler published *The Conquest of Cancer*. She warned her readers not to eat chicken or eggs:

> "After years of research, I consider the potential for cancer in chicken to be almost one hundred percent. Most of the chickens on the dining tables of America have the pathogenic form of the microbe, which I contend is transmissable to human beings."

She called for vaccinating cattle and chicken with the anti-cancer serum. Rife had long envisioned using the Rife Ray to kill the BX in chickens and meat. He also had specifically warned that BX (cancer) virus thrived on pig and mushrooms. The wheel kept turning and turning.

When it is realized that the disease-causing micro-organisms in food can be devitalized, and that the blood in hospital blood banks may need to be similarly purified, the loss of Rife's discovery can be seen in its true tragic dimensions.

Dr. Livingston-Wheeler also called for cancer immunization soon after the birth of every child (the serum can be made from a urine sample). She knew the signs of a cancer epidemic were everywhere if anyone bothered to look. She also declared that cancer could be permanently wiped out in a decade. Rife had known how to do it also . . . but in a country where 60 billion dollars are spent annually on cancer, where one tiny hospital in the Berkshires of Massachusetts can spend 2½ million dollars for "state-of-the-art" radiation equipment, it is clear that an entire economy of satisfied cancer "professionals" exists, determined to keep their gruesome racket in place.

Dr. Livingston-Wheeler's book was completed on July 23, 1983 in La Jolla. Forty-nine years earlier at the Scripps Ranch in La Jolla, a man staggered onto a table with cancer so bad that when doctors felt his stomach they could almost touch his backbone. In a few months time, he was driving his car and staying up all night with a sick cow. Cancer could be cured. Cancer *had* been cured.

Chapter 17

The Victims

Perhaps a word here about the human victims is needed. Statistics don't tell the true story of what individual human beings suffered because Roy Rife's discoveries were suppressed, because the AMA was guarding its pocket book, because the pharmaceutical companies had "chemotherapy" to push for profit, because the American Cancer Society was a big money public relations fraud, because the FDA was owned by the cancer monopolies, because the media was silent, silent, silent.

Two accounts tell the tale. These stories can be multiplied by millions and millions.

Dorothy Lynch of Dorchester, Massachusetts died of cancer. She tried so hard to learn about alternative therapies. But the cancer establishment pushed her into all the traditional methods. Dorothy wrote a book about her long, terrible voyage through the cancer wards. Her husband Eugene Richards took pictures of her during the ordeal and also pictures of others on the same hellish path. *Exploding Into Life* is a visual and word portrait showing how Fishbein, Rivers, Rhoads, the bosses of the American Cancer Society—and all the cowards who might have stood up but didn't—have murdered and maimed.

The other cancer book which is a testament to America's holocaust is *The Great Planet Swap and Other Stories*. It was written by 9 year old Mark Johnson of La Crosse, Wisconsin. It includes stories of a boy with cancer and his hospital experiences until he finally went home. Only Mark didn't go home. He died of leukemia after "battling" it and the chemotherapy for 4 years. The tale of the I. V. "toobs," shots and radiation is perhaps America's sequel to *The Diary of Anne Frank*.

These deaths did not have to happen. Dorothy and Mark could have led normal, happy lives. In 1953, a naval officer who had known Roy Rife when the officer was a young man growing up in San Diego wrote Rife a letter. He explained how in his military career he commanded a unit of doctors and bacteriologists. The letter is a fitting epitaph to the Rife tragedy:

"I have been very privileged in having known you and having heard from your own lips the story of your work. You gave me a glimpse of science of the year 2000. But often I'm a little sad when I realize that men must struggle so hard to get what you tried to give them, and I am even more sad when I see so many problems for which you alone have the answers. When I see pictures taken with the electron microscope, I have to laugh, because I remember better pictures showing more detail which were hung in the hallway in your laboratory. When I read 'research' reports on genetics, evolution, or any of the fields of microbiology I have to laugh, because years ago the 'scientists' were offered the answers and they refused the gift! The combination of your mind, your will, and your energy is so rare as to skip entire generations. The world has great need for your work.

"Perhaps the world will someday rediscover one of the greatest gifts on which it has ever turned its back. Someday we may develop equipment similar to the Rife Ray machine. If and when that happens, our problems will be solved. Man will have more food and structural materials than he needs. For the first time the economic reasons for wars will cease to exist. By then, the AMA will be forced to accept its use for the elimination of disease organisms. Man will live a healthier, happier and longer life.

"If we reach that millenium in my life, I will have one unhappy memory—that the man most deserving to have his name linked for all time with human happiness will have been all but forgotten because his life's work was lost in a struggle with the AMA and the 'accepted' scientists of his day rather than made available through a new approach; and because when it is rediscovered, the Rife Ray will be given a new name."

Chapter 18
Clarifications and Explanations
(Added 1997, ten years after the original publication)

A decade ago I wrote the book you are now reading. I never imagined then that the medical bosses, scientific elite, and government health agencies that so totally suppressed Rife for half a century would retain that control for another ten years. But changes are in the wind. A vast alternative health movement is afoot, even though the barricades around the old guard "cancer experts" remain formidable. There is now overwhelming evidence of the damage inflicted by conventional cancer treatments on a trusting, innocent, essentially brainwashed cancer patient "market." A lot of money is being made through a very evil, highly unyielding system.

"As a chemist trained to interpret data, it is incomprehensible to me that physicians can ignore the clear evidence that chemotherapy does much, much more harm than good."

Alan C. Nixon, Ph.D., Past President, Amer. Chem. Soc.; quoted in *Questioning Chemotherapy*, by Ralph Moss

Rife's incredible, unique microscope and his pioneering discoveries in "energy medicine" or "wave-form medicine" or "resonance healing" (all modern terms) will have their place in a very different 21st century medicine. And Rife, I am certain, will eventually gain his deserved place in medical history, once the current "Berlin Wall" of orthodox cancer treatment comes crashing down.

Until that happens, I believe it is important to clear up a few misconceptions which orthodox scientists, doctors, and bureaucrats use to dismiss Rife's great work.

"The ages cannot kill a truth, and the first man who phrased it will find his echo right down through the centuries."

Paul Brunton

What Rife saw in his microscope, and isolated as one cause if not the cause for many cancers, was a *microbe*. A cancer microbe. Keep that in mind. It is crucial to understanding the tremendous implications of Rife's great accomplishment for the medical science of tomorrow.

A microbe is a catch-all term. We still do not know what Rife's BX was. A virus? A "dwarf" bacterium? Some transitional form? Scientists of the 1990s are uncertain whether viruses are even alive. They now have *viroids* and *P-Viruses* as well as "normal" viruses. So don't be fooled. If you encounter a quick dismissal of Rife, ask about the inability of modern science to cure cancer. That is the crucial issue. All else is hocus-pocus.

Resonance, at its own frequency, is a property of everything on earth, which is why Rife could cure cancer, be its cause a true virus, a "dwarf bacterium", or something in between!

Bacteria are single-cell organisms, many of which cause terrible diseases. Antibiotics attack bacteria by breaking through the bacterial *cell wall*. But many bacteria have, through mutation, become resistant to antibiotics. Antibiotic abuse by patients and overprescribing by physicians may be ushering the world's population into a perilous place where old and terrible or new and terrible diseases, caused by bacteria, are a constant threat. Any honest medical scientist will admit this!

Size: "A typical bacterium... measures about... 1/25,000 of an inch... a large virus... is about one quarter that large... A single virus ranges from about .01 to .3 microns in diameter... as little as two millionths of an inch across." (Peter Radetsky, *The Invisible Invaders*, 1991.

A virus is a wad of DNA or RNA surrounded by a protein coat. According to official science, a bacterium cannot change into a virus or vice-versa. Fine. But that's not the critical issue. Rife's *cancer microbe* caused cancer (he used Koch's historic postulates to prove it!) and Rife cured it in mice and in humans by painlessly destroying his four *cancer microbes* -- the BX, BY, fungus, and large round coccoid forms.

Turning a blind eye: The refusal to investigate Rife's cancer healing treatment "in earnest" remains one of the great crimes of this

124

century. "*In earnest* in contemporary research largely means money." (Ann Giudici Fettner, *The Science of Viruses*, 1990, page 117.)

What autopsies show: "I studied autopsies of...patients who had been treated with massive doses of antibiotics for weeks before death: the antibiotics failed to kill the cancer microbes. I saw the microbe in tissues that had been burned with massive doses of radiation....I saw the microbe thriving in cancerous tissue that had been blitzed with chemotherapy; the cancer cells were destroyed, but the...microbe remained! Nothing fazed the cancer microbe: not surgery, not radiation, not antibiotics, not chemotherapy..." (Alan Cantwell, Jr., M.D., *The Cancer Microbe*, 1990, p. 115.)

What Rife did: "Royal Rife...examined cancers with the optical microscopes which he designed and built...he then designed...electrical machines which he could tune to certain frequencies and apparently cause the viruses to disintegrate as he observed them with his microscope..." (Peter Macomber, M.D., Harvard-trained pathologist and former Asst. Chief of Experimental Pathology at Walter Reed Army Institute of Pathology, Washington, D.C., from *Townsend Letter for Doctors*, Oct 1994.)

Suppression continued: By the mid-1960s, official science had recognized the "something" which Rife's M.O.R. approach and super microscope, in combination, were able to destroy. But for 30 years more, the guardians of orthodox medicine at the FDA, the National Cancer Institute, the AMA, the "big league" cancer hospitals and research universities, the all-powerful *New Englsnd Journal of Medicine*, the media, and the United States Congress have kept Rife's discoveries from desperate cancer patients...to the ever-lasting shame of the officials of these institutions.

Compare the following description from a mid-1960s book on microbes (*The World of Microbes*, edited by Alan Delaunay, Doubleday Pub., 1965, page 43) with what Rife was doing 30 years earlier, and better, and curing cancer as a result:

"... there appear granulations, called 'dwarf forms', of very small dimensions, measuring in fact a millionth of a millimetre... They seem to be rather fragile and possess a very special property, due to their smallness, of being able to go through the walls of filters

125

which retain normal bacteria... The experimentor, by adding substances to a culture, has been able to transform a bacterium of normal dimensions, non-filterable and reproducing by fission, into another form, difficult to see, of much smaller dimensions, filterable, and which reproduces by an altogether different mechanism."

A personal note: It took me years to realize that the people in control of the cancer treatment world *today* did not want a simple, quick cure for cancer. It was not in their economic or *career* interest. They wanted complicated disease syndromes and all the paraphernalia of techniques, expert analyses, peer group conferences, papers, discussions, research grants and clinical trials *for years* before a new cancer therapy might be allowed. It is a horrendous crime which serves only those "inside" who are playing the great, lucrative "expert" game. No matter whether the treatment was Rife's, Hulda Clark's, Mildred Nelson's, Rene Caisse's, Kelley's, Gregory's, Ozone, or lots of others.

Meanwhile, there existed tons of money for constructing medical "white elephants." Buildings, yes! Honest testing of cancer cures for the sake of millions of cancer patients? No!

"The hospitals in New York State are among the financially sickest in the nation... Yet for several years, these same hospitals have been able to go on building sprees. They have pursued huge projects, some costing hundreds of millions of dollars, to erect gleaming inpatient palaces in the sky." (Lucette Lagnado, *Wall Street Journal*, November 22, 1996, p. 1.)

By 1939-1940, the electron microscope had enabled "official" science to *see* viruses. In 1949 John Enders opened the "Age of Viruses" when he discovered how to cultivate viruses in laboratory tissue cultures. An explosion of research followed into the world Rife was studying decades before! Yet when Rife's energy medicine approach to disabling the cancer microbe was attempted again in the 1950s... Well, the original book published in 1987 picks up this tragic tale once more in Chapter 19...

How The Legal System Was Corrupted To Suppress Rife's Cancer Cure

In this book we have seen (1) how Roy Rife invented a super microscope which enabled scientists to see viruses in their live state and "stain" the viruses with color instead of chemicals; (2) how Roy Rife invented Frequency Instruments (FI) which, using electronic frequencies set on the unique rate of each virus, destroyed them in slides, in animals, and in humans; (3) how medical, pharmaceutical, cancer and political authorities combined to suppress the discovery and its various techniques.

What has *not* yet been covered in this book is that in 1950 Rife became partners with John Crane, with the result that the microscope and Frequency Instruments were not only improved and further developed through a cooperative effort, but re-invented according to a new design of John Crane's. What happened to John Crane provides a sad footnote to the Rife story. The reader is warned. It will shock those who believe that the American legal system prevents abuse of the little man by the "powers that be." If ever there were grounds for the American Bar Association, the American Congress, and the media to investigate a miscarriage of justice, it is here, in the story of John Crane.

In 1950, John Crane met Roy Rife. After learning how Rife had cured cancer in the 1930s but had seen his cure suppressed by the AMA, Crane decided to commit his energy, will and electronic and mechanical knowledge to bringing the cure for cancer to the public. Dr. Gruner of Canada, who worked with Rife in the '30s, provided Crane with one of the original circuit designs for the Rife Ray Tube. Crane also hired Verne Thomson, an electronics expert with the San Diego police force, to help construct the new Frequency Instruments.

In April 1953, the first copyrighted material on the cancer virus was published. In December 1953, Rife's description of the cancer cure was completed under Crane's urging and insistence. It was copyrighted in 1954.

In 1954, Crane began corresponding with the National Cancer Institute and other government agencies concerning the Rife diagnostic and therapeutic instruments. In 1954, the Committee on Cancer Diagnosis and Therapy of the National Research Council "evaluated" the Rife discoveries. They concluded it couldn't work. No effort was made to contact Rife, Gruner, Couche or others who had witnessed actual cures (Couche was still curing cancer patients at that time). No physical inspection of the instruments was attempted. Electronic healing was bureaucratically determined to be impossible. (In 1972, Carl G. Baker, M.D., Director of the National Cancer Institute, used this superficial 1954 evaluation to dismiss Crane's and Rife's work when asked for information by Congressman Bob Wilson of San Diego. Millions died and continue to die because government and medical authorities were opposed to a fair, objective evaluation of the evidence.)

While working on the Frequency Instrument from 1954 to 1957, Crane slowly began to get results. Each improvement brought him closer to his goal: curing cancer. Rife continued to aid him, but in essence the two men were now working together and discovering together. Because neither had the resources which were available to Rife in the 1930s, building a high powered Ray Tube was impossible. But Crane thought he could do just as well with a much smaller Frequency Instrument which attached to the body during treatment. This is exactly what evolved.

In 1957, Crane made contact with Dr. Robert Stafford of Dayton, Ohio. Stafford was interested in using the Frequency Instrument both in clinical treatment and in new laboratory tests on mice. By November 1957, Stafford had 6 months of testing behind him. His initial evaluation was positive. Of 4 person with cancer, one made "remarkable and unexpected improvement." The other three were treated while in a terminal stage. All died, but all obtained relief once the treatment was initiated. Two were autopsied. The results showed they had died from other causes. There was a "surprising paucity of cancer cells." Stafford also noted that of 33 patients treated for a variety of ailments, *none* experienced any detrimental effects from the treatments.

Then, in 1958, Crane made his great breakthrough. He made another in 1960, enabling hundreds of times more energy to be concentrated on the deadly virus. These methods have never been published and are the heart of Crane's legitimate patent claims.

By February 1958, Dr. Stafford in Dayton, Ohio had presented his findings to the Executive Committee of the General Practice Section of the Montgomery County Medical Society of the A.M.A. The 8 doctors were impressed. Stafford began setting up a Research Committee with Dayton's most influential doctors. If the anti-Rife forces hadn't crushed Crane a few years later, much might have been accomplished in Dayton where objective evaluation was being offered.

In early 1958, doctors in Salt Lake City, Utah also began using the Frequency Instrument. But in May 1958, the Salt Lake County Medical Board forced them to stop using the electronic treatment. One of the cancer patients broke down and "wept bitterly when the doctor had to tell him he could not continue the treatments." The same doctor later told an associate in Salt Lake City that "if his own family had cancer— he would immediately purchase a machine and use it on his own family. This would indicate how sold he must be." The writer of the letter concluded, "Too many people have been saying things that have aroused the ire of the medical profession here." It was an old story—a re-run of California in the late '30s when the medical profession suddenly saw their authority and incomes threatened.

1958 also brought a hearing before the state of California Public Health Department. A Frequency Instrument was provided and tested by the Palo Alto Detection Lab, the Kalbfeld Lab, the UCLA Medical Lab, and the San Diego Testing Lab. All reported it was *safe to use*. Nevertheless, the AMA board under the Director of Public Health Dr. Malcolm Merrill declared it *unsafe* and banned it from the market.

Still, despite the setback, Crane continued toward his and

Rife's goal. By February, Dr. Stafford in Dayton suggested that he, Stafford, manufacture and distribute the Frequency Instruments in the Eastern United States. He contacted a qualified electrical engineer, obtained a patent attorney, and began canvassing for venture capital. Obviously, the results he was seeing in his hospital and with experimental mice were convincing.

Crane decided to license the machines in order to prevent doctors from changing the instrument and thus failing to get results—Rife's experience with Dr. Yale and Hoyland being the example. Since Crane already had completed a preliminary patent application with a California patent attorney, he sent it to Dr. Stafford for the Ohio patent attorney to examine. The two patent attorneys agreed "all was in order."

However, they couldn't submit it to the government patent office until the "usefulness" of the invention could be shown. Thus, they held back work until enough doctors and others experimenting with the different frequencies could provide substantial evidence. With no organized medical, scientific and laboratory involvement in the research—as had existed in the '30s—Crane and Rife were forced to establish "usefulness" under a terribly difficult handicap. Opposition from the California Public Health Department and the experience in Salt Lake City, not to mention the AMA assault in 1939, meant they were in a "Catch-22" situation regarding patenting.

So Crane leased the Frequency Instrument in order to build his experimental base and thus prove the "usefulness" of his invention. The numbers of people who were being healed began to mount. He slowly gathered reports, testimonials and evidence. He refined his procedures for training new operators. As in 1938, the *breakout* point was nearing.

By 1960, Crane had written and copyrighted a manual which explained how the Frequency Instrument was to be used in the experimental treatment of various diseases and on different parts of the body. By that year, 90 instruments were distributed for research and verification on notarized contracts. And then the medical authorities struck.

They raided Crane's office, took over $40,000 in machines, frequency instruments, and one large Rife ray tube instrument, along with engineering data, research records and reports, pictures off the wall, private letters, invoices, tape recordings, and electronic parts—all without a search warrant.

They smashed all the research which had been put together over 10 laborious years. As in 1939, they visited the doctors who were experimenting with the machines and forced them to abandon them. They also pressured ordinary citizens who had begun experimenting on a personal basis.

These visits were made by teams of investigators. "One woman was scared so bad that she has been in a sanitarium driven entirely out of her mind. Her husband cursed them out and told them to get off his property and has threatened to exterminate them should they return. His wife has undergone shock treatments and two months of hospitalization."

The records and materials seized were not allowed to be used by Crane in his own defense during his trial.

Roy Rife, almost 73 and incapable of suffering the abuse of another trial at his age, went into hiding in Mexico. *His deposition was not permitted to be introduced at the trial.* Neither were the medical and scientific reports from the 1930s and 1940s. Nor were medical reports from Dr. Stafford in Ohio. Dr. Couche's letters were also declared inadmissable. No medical or scientific report which indicated the Frequency Instrument worked as represented was permitted to be introduced at the trial. Crane was left naked with only the patients who had been cured or helped.

The trial was held in early 1961. After 24 days, and despite the testimony of 14 patients who told how the Frequency Instrument cured ailments and diseases which orthodox medicine could not alleviate, Crane was found guilty. The only medical opinion offered by the State of California came from Dr. Paul Shea who had been given a Frequency Instrument by the Public Health Department for 2 months before the trial. Shea admitted he never tried the Frequency Instrument on anything or made any tests to evaluate it. He simply examined it and decided that it had no curative powers and didn't lend itself to investigative use.

Also, and most disturbing, the foreman of the jury was an AMA doctor. Everyone else was carefully screened to see that they had no medical knowledge, no electronic knowledge, and didn't read any newspapers supporting alternative healing. The verdict was a foregone conclusion. Crane was sentenced to 10 years in jail. Following appeals, two of the three counts against Crane were reversed in the California Supreme Court because no specific criminal intent had been proven. But Crane still spent 3 years and 1 month in jail. The cure for cancer had been effectively suppressed again.

During the trial, James Hannibal, age 76, testified. Blind in one eye, he'd been treated by the Frequency Instrument. After several applications, his cataract disappeared—just as cataracts had dissolved in many of Dr. Milbank Johnson's patients during the 1935-37 clinics. Other witnesses at Crane's trial testified to the curing of chronic bladder irritation, and the elimination of a throat lump one-half of the size of an egg. Also cured were fungus growths on hands, fissures in the anus, pyorrhea, arthritis, ulcerated colon, varicose veins, prostrate troubles, tumorous growth over eyes, colitis, pains in the back, and heart attacks. One man testified that for 17 years he had a growth the size of an egg on his spine. After treatment, it had disappeared.

After Crane was imprisoned, so much pressure was put on Dr. Stafford in Ohio that he gave up medicine and became a salesman. Another doctor in Salt Lake City had his Frequency Instrument sabotaged and then was hounded by the orthodox medical authorities to such an extent that he committed suicide. Such were the lengths to which the anti-Rife forces were willing to go in order to prevent the testing and use of this breakthrough technology.

When Crane was released from prison, the cure for cancer was in shambles. A weaker man might have thrown in the towel. But Crane didn't waiver. He started to fight all over again. With little money and no legal help, he began a seemingly hopeless campaign to keep alive the discoveries which had been persecuted and denied to the public since the 1930s.

In October 1965, Crane submitted an application to the California Board of Public Health, seeking approval of the Frequency Instrument. Rife was back from Mexico but hanging in the background. The application was made in the name of Rife Virus Microscope Institute of which John Crane was the owner. On November 17, 1965, the Department of Public Health replied that Crane had not shown that the device was safe or "effective in use." Again, Crane could not prove to the authorities that the Frequency Instrument's "usefulness" was a fact. Although the reports from the 1930s and the limited research in the late 1950s clearly demonstrated that extraordinary healing results had occurred, nonetheless without living authorities willing to put their expertise and medical licenses on the line, the state officials wouldn't approve it. But every time doctors, researchers and ordinary citizens got to the point where the validation of "usefulness" seemed near, the medical authorities quashed further research. Crane and Rife could not patent their great medical discovery without proving "usefulness." They couldn't interest financial men and researchers without "usefulness." And the medical authorities and public officials' deadly game had a parallel death count for innocent citizens—hundreds of thousands per year as the paper went back and forth.

Crane attempted to respond to the Department of Health's request for proof of "usefulness." Dr. Charles W. Bunner, a Chiropractor, was one of the men who agreed to provide a statement about the Frequency Instrument's effectiveness. As soon as he did, the same Department of Health which requested such "proof" from Crane paid a visit to Dr. Bunner. They forbade him from using his Frequency Instrument and then a court ordered it "destroyed." Such was justice in mid-1960s California. Such was objective medical evaluation.

The second man to provide a statement to the California Department of Health was Dr. Les Drown, also a Chiropractor. An employee of the American Cancer Society was soon sent to Dr. Drown's office to entrap him. He was forced to "sign over" his Frequency Instrument or go to jail.

Rife and Crane were intending to patent their joint microscope in the late 1950s along with the Frequency Instrument. A microscope diagram for patenting purposes was drafted with both names listed as inventors. Rife also was intending to patent his Universal Microscope. The assault on the cancer cure in 1960 disrupted their plans. Without being able to show

133

"usefulness," Rife and Crane could not patent their discoveries. The actions by the defenders of medical orthodoxy stymied every attempt Rife and Crane made to bring the cure for cancer to the general public.

Rife had obtained a patent on a microscope lamp in 1929, but that was before the threat he represented to the orthodox medical (and scientific) establishment was recognized. By the middle and late '60s, Rife had witnessed or learned about: (1) the spectacle of the AMA crushing his discoveries in 1939 and forcing doctors to abandon them even when numerous cancer cures were on record; (2) the mysterious death of Dr. Milbank Johnson in 1944, apparently just when he was preparing to make an announcement about cancer being curable; (3) the strange theft of the prism from the Universal Microscope just after the article on the microscope and curing cancer appeared in the Smithsonian Institution report; (4) the hopeful revitalization of the 1950s under Crane's direction—crushed in the 1960 travesty of justice when all research was confiscated and scientific reports were forbidden to be introduced at the trial; and (5) the mid-1960s attempt at legitimization and the way the medical authorities again had pressured researchers and health practitioners to quit.

Rife would be 80 years in May 1968. He had fought his last war. He knew he was unlikely to see his Frequency Instruments or his microscopes used to heal virus-caused diseases. And he was uncertain about the protracted exchanges with the Patent Office which lay ahead, especially when the issue of "usefulness" was a Catch-22 situation for which there was no obvious solution. Medical treatment had to be approved by medical and scientific authorities. Every time such men appeared and offered Rife and Crane help, the medical powers crushed them or forced them to give up Rife-associated research or treatment.

So on March 4, 1968, Royal R. Rife signed ownership of his microscope over to John F. Crane, indicating that he intended to patent it and that John Crane would own all rights. Rife considered the Frequency Instruments to be joint inventions because of all the original work that both Rife and Crane had done on them.

It is important that John Crane's contribution in keeping alive Rife's work be recognized. Crane preserved the records and never quit when the going got tough, as many others did. But it is also important to acknowledge that Crane was in many ways inadequate to the task he assumed. He did not have the management or political skills which Dr. Milbank Johnson had demonstrated, and was not able to "bring aboard" the qualified scientists, businessmen, financiers and attorneys who could have altered the course of medical history.

Unfortunately, Crane managed to antagonize many of the professionals who offered help, and his efforts to legitimize the Rife instruments in the 1950s were not as professional as they might have been.

Crane bore the brunt of the medical, political and legal opposition to the Rife legacy, and he became bitter. He wasted years filing ill-advised lawsuits against the State of California, Vice President Nelson Rockefeller and some fifty-two other persons and organizations. Acting as his own lawyer, Crane launched attacks that were a mishmash of accusations and citations. While the cases dragged on, hundreds of thousands continued to die every year.

In 1959, a year before the authorities struck, Crane was demanding $150 million from interested investors—an unusually high amount for the time. Interested investors apparently existed, but they evidently did not view Crane as a person to whom serious seed money should be advanced, no matter how brilliant or profitable Rife's scientific genius.

Following Rife's death in 1971, Crane continued to attract interested investors, but no agreements were concluded.

From 1984 to 1988, Rife's Universal Microscope passed through the hands of several groups and individuals who undertook to restore it, but no progress was made toward this goal. A federal legal action had to be initiated in order to have it returned, finally, to its legitimate owners—Rife Labs, a company formed to revitalize Rife's work in accordance with modern scientific methods.

John Crane died in the spring of 1995. A great deal of the failure to resurrect Rife's discoveries and inventions in a way which would bring them into mainstream acceptance and utilization for countless people can be attributed to Crane's greed, ego and obstructionism. He and a cohort of cronies, crooks and low-lifes who surrounded him during the period 1987-1995 tried to exploit this book for their own gain, in a way which not only did not serve the larger public interest, but utterly failed (indeed, did not even attempt) to corroborate Rife's findings.

Fortunately, by 1996, a new breed of Rife-inspired, energy "resonance" medicine pioneers was emerging. The future of this revolutionary approach to healing many diseases and vitalizing people to new heights of health appears very hopeful.

Crane died with a reputation for dishonest dealings. He had given the world a precious gift—preserving Rife's accomplishment—but he apparently never comprehended his own greater obligations, and could not rise above his own narrow self-interest in order to accomplish objectives which clearly could have been attained through righteous dealings.

And yet, as the 21st Century began, Rife's work was very much "alive" again in the world, on the internet and elsewhere, spreading, with Rife's spirit radiating anew, with "resonance healing" coming on like the Dawn's revivifying RAYS. The future could blaze with Rife-related breakthroughs!

Selected Bibliography

Annals of the New York Academy of Sciences, Vol. 174, October 30, 1970.

Beale, Morris: *Super Drug Story.* Columbia Pub., Washington, D.C., 1949.

———: *Medical Mussolini.* Columbia Pub., Washington, D.C., 1939.

Benison, Tom: *Tom Rivers: Reflection on a Life in Medicine and Science.* MIT Press, Cambridge, Ma., 1967.

Bird, Christopher: "What Has Become of the Rife Microscope?" *New Age Journal.* Boston, March 1976.

Brown, Raymond K.: *AIDS, Cancer and the Medical Establishment.* Aries Rising Press, Los Angeles, 1986.

Cantwell, Alan, Jr.: *AIDS: The Mystery and the Solution.* Aries Rising Press, Los Angeles, 1983.

Corner, George: *History of Rockefeller Institute 1901-1953.* Rockefeller Institute Press, New York, 1964.

Crane, John: *A Study of Electron Therapy.* John F. Crane Corp., San Diego, 1978.

Cullen, Ben, transcript of interview, October 15, 1959.

Dominigue, Gerald J.: *Cell-Wall Deficient Bacteria.* Addison-Wesley, Reading, Ma., 1982.

"Filtrable Bodies Seen With The Rife Microscope," *Science-Supplement, Science,* December 11, 1931.

"Giant Microscope May Yield Secrets of Bacteria World," *Los Angeles Times,* June 26, 1940.

Gruner, O.C.: *Study of Blood in Cancer.* Renouf, Montreal, 1942.

"Here Is Most Powerful Microscope," *Los Angeles Times*, November 27, 1931.

Hoyland vs. Beam Ray Corp., June 12, 1939, Judge Edward Kelly presiding, transcript, San Diego.

Hume, E. Douglas: *Bechamp or Pasteur*. C. W. Daniel Co., Ltd., Essex, 1947.

Jones, Newell, "Dread Disease Germs Destroyed by Rays Claim of S. D. Scientist," *San Diego Tribune*, May 6, 1938.

Jones, Newell, "Rife Bares Startling New Conceptions of Disease Germs," *San Diego Tribune*, May 11, 1938.

Keller, Evelyn F.: *A Feeling For The Organism*. W. H. Freeman & Co., San Francisco, 1983.

Kendall, Arthur & Rife, Royal, "Observations on Bacillus Typhosus in its Filtrable State," *California and Western Medicine*, December 1931.

Kendall, Arthur, "The Filtration of Bacteria," *Science*, March 18, 1932.

Livingston-Wheeler, Virginia and Addeo, Edmund G.: *The Conquest of Cancer*. Franklin Watts, 1984.

"Local Man Bares Wonders of Germ Life," *San Diego Union*. November 3, 1929.

Locke, David: *Viruses—The Smallest Enemy*. Crown Pub., New York, 1974.

Mattman, Lida H.: *Cell Wall Deficient Forms*. CRC Press, Cleveland, Ohio, 1974.

Moss, Ralph: *The Cancer Syndrome*. Grove Press, New York, 1980.

Natenberg, Maurice: *The Cancer Blackout*. Regent House, Chicago, 1959.

National Cyclopedia of American Biography, Vol. 49 (Kendall). James T. White and Co., New York, 1966.

Nicholas, Robin and Nicholas, David: *Virology, An Information Profile*. Mansell Pub., London, 1983.

Ransome, _____, "What's New In Science—The Wonderwork of 1931," *Los Angeles Times Sunday Magazine*, December 27, 1931.

Rife Microscope or Facts and their Fate. Reprint #47, The Lee Foundation for Nutritional Research, Milwaukee, Wi.

Rife, Royal R.: *History of the Development of a Successful Treatment for Cancer and Other Virus, Bacteria and Fungi.* Rife Virus Microscope Institute, San Diego, Ca., 1953.

————, Documents and Correspondence, 1920-71.

Rosenow, E. C., "Transmutations Within the Streptococcus-Pneumococcus Group," *Journal of Infectious Diseases,* Vol. 14, 1914.

————, "Observations on Filter-Passing Forms of Streptococcus from Poliomelitis," *Proceedings of the Staff Meetings of the Mayo Clinic,* 13 July 1932.

————, "Observations with the Rife Microscope of Filter-Passing Forms of Microorganisms," *Science.* August 26, 1932.

"Science's Latest Strides in War on Ills Disclosed, Development by San Diegan Hailed as Boon to Medical Research," *Los Angeles Times,* November 22, 1931.

Seibert, Florence B.: *Pebbles on the Hill of a Scientist.* St. Petersburg, Fl., 1968.

Seidel, R. E. and Winter, M. Elizabeth, "The New Microscopes," *Journal of the Franklin Institute,* February 1944.

Sonea, Sorin & Panisset, Maurice: *A New Bacteriology.* Jones & Bartlett, Boston, 1983.

Starr, Paul: *The Social Transformation of American Medicine.* Basic Books, New York, 1982.

"Virus Found 15 Years Ago—San Diegan's Cancer Cure Work May Make Cure Possible," *San Diego Union,* July 31, 1949.

Wuerthele-Caspe, Virginia and Allen, Roy, *New York Microscopical Society Bulletin,* August 1948.

Wuerthele-Caspe, Virginia, *American Journal of Medical Sciences,* December 1950.

Wuerthele-Caspe-Livingston, Virginia: *Cancer, A New Breakthrough.* Nash Pub., Los Angeles, 1972.

Yale, Arthur W., "Cancer," *Pacific Coast Journal of Homeopathy,* July 1940.

List of Appendices

A. Johnson to Rife, November 1931
B. Photo of the doctors' gathering, November 1931
C. News clipping photo of Rife, December 1931
D. Rife's cancer notes, November 1932
E. Johnson to Rife, September 1933 (Foord)
F. Rife's 1933 article
G. Photograph of the Universal Microscope, built in 1933
H. Rife's notes, February 1934 (Foord)
I. Johnson to Rife, April 1934 (clinic plans)
J. Rife's description of the 1934 clinic
K. Cancer virus characteristics
L. Kendall Letter, September 1934 (Tom Knight)
M. Johnson to Rife, March 1935 (Cancer Foundation)
N. Johnson to Rife, May 1935 (Mrs. Young's TB)
O. Johnson to Rife, September 1935 (Foord and Dock)
P. Johnson to Rife, October 1935 (Committee's legal releases)
Q. Johnson to Rife, December 1935 (Committee meeting)
R. Johnson to Rife, January 1937 (Dock & Martin)
S. Rife and his microscope, October 1940
T. Dr. Tully's statement, June 1954
U. Rife in his laboratory (picture) 1960
V. Dr. Chromiak's statement, January 1965
W. Affidavit of cured cancer victim, January 1968
X. Research summary of bacteria/virus characteristics

Appendix A

MILBANK JOHNSON, M. D.
PACIFIC MUTUAL LIFE BLDG.
LOS ANGELES, CALIFORNIA

November 9, 1931

My dear Mr. Rife:

In the name of the other three gentlemen and myself I want to thank you for your most courteous reception and for giving us an opportunity to have a glance of your wonderful microscope. I want to say to you that we all spent one of the most instructive and interesting afternoons of our lives in your laboratory.

Upon returning to San Diego that evening I wired to Dr. Arthur I. Kendall of Chicago and gave him a brief description of what we had seen and our opinion of it, and upon my return to Pasadena this morning I received the following telegram from Dr. Kendall - "Expect to start for California Saturday night. Letter follows".

If he comes straight through, which I think he will, he will arrive in Pasadena on Tuesday, November 17 so be sure and have your microscope in perfect condition for the Big Chief when he arrives. I will bring him down to San Diego in my car at which time you and Dr. Kendall can make such arrangements as you desire.

Thanking you again for your courtesy, I am

Yours very sincerely,

Milbank Johnson

600 BURLEIGH DRIVE
SAN RAFAEL HEIGHTS
PASADENA

Mr. Roy Rife
2500 Chatsworth Bldg.
San Diego, Calif.

143

Appendix B

The Doctor's Gathering—Nov 1931

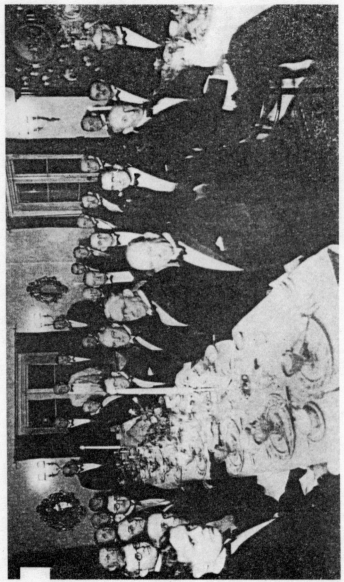

Kendall, Johnson & Rife are in front of the window

Appendix C

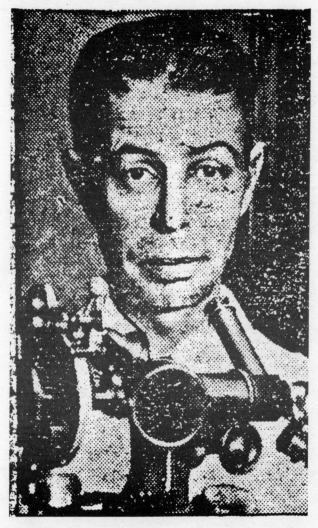

Royal Raymond Rife has perfected a microscope said by Pasadena scientists to be the most powerful in the world. It magnifies to 17,000 diameters.

Appendix D

Bacillus X (Cancer) Carcinoma
(Rife) 11-20-32

Filterable Virus: Passes W: K Medium

motile small ovoid granule
highly plastic
visable only with mono chromatic light
angle of refraction   12³/10
color by chemical refraction Purple-red
length - 1/15 u :: breadth 1/20 u.

Polarity
        + anode
        - cathode   X
Death rate in milliamperes 175 D.C.
Influence of X rays   none
    "   " Ultra Violet ray slows motility
    "   " Infra Red   none
Thermal death point   42C. 24 hrs.
Filament voltage   10
    "   amperage   86
Plate voltage   928
Cycles per second   11,780,000
Wave length of super regeneration of audien tube 17 3/10 met.

146

Appendix E

MILBANK JOHNSON, M.D.
PACIFIC MUTUAL LIFE BLDG.
LOS ANGELES, CALIFORNIA

September 5, 1933

My dear Dr. Rife,

I mailed you this morning from
Pasadena a letter just received from
Dr. Kendall which is self-explanatory.

It is very evident now that this
sleeping sickness which has been so
prevalent in St. Louis has appeared in
Chicago. Dr. Kendall says in this letter
that he wishes that he could have you and
your microscope with him to make examinations
of cultures, spinal fluid, and blood with a
view to isolating this germ for which
everybody is seeking.

You two would make a wonderful
combination and any germ that escapes your
eagle eye would certainly be a small one.
I am sending you this letter because you may
hear from him direct and you will know what
it is all about.

Yours sincerely,

Milbank Johnson

Dr. Royal R. Rife
2500 Chatsworth Blvd.
San Diego, Calif.

P.S. Dr. Foord has finished the study of the pig – has
written a full report, & made sections which he says
that he will send you in a few days –

MJ

600 BURLEIGH DRIVE
SAN RAFAEL HEIGHTS
PASADENA

147

Appendix F

Viruses and Rickettsia of Certain Diseases (1933)

By Royal R. Rife

It is the purpose of this paper to give a brief resume of the reports on file in our laboratory dealing with virus experimentation and also to treat on the etiological significance of the Rickettsia Bodies in connection with certain diseases.

The existing theories regarding the viruses are entirely unsatisfactory and sadly wanting of further elucidation. Therefore, we shall expound our theories at the outset with the hope that other workers may find them sufficiently basic to serve as an incentive for checking our observations.

The virus diseases of plants and animals are probably caused by organisms exhibiting certain transitional stages in a cycle under given conditions. All of the viruses are fully virulent after they have been passed through certain diatomaceous earth or porcelain filters. The filterability of these bodies alone does not serve as a means of classifying them. They must also exhibit other important properties before they can be considered in the category of virus bodies.

Most of the known viruses exist only in close association with the living cells of the host. Many attempts have been made to cultivate them on artificial media, but with little success.

The writer has long entertained the assumption that it is possible to cultivate viruses on artificial media. After many failures on my own behalf, it was my privilege and good fortune to work with Dr. Arthur Isaac Kendall of Northwestern University Medical School on the problem of culturing viruses under artificial conditions, using his protein-rich, peptone-poor, "K" Medium. The successful results obtained in our initial experiments are on record in a joint publication by Dr. Kendall and myself which appeared in California and Western Medicine, Volume XXXV, No. 6. The importance of that work was indicated in a later report that was published in Proceedings of the Staff Meetings of the Mayo Clinic, Volume 7, No. 28, by E. C. Rosenow, M. D., Division of Experimental Bacteriology. In this report were recorded the more important observations made during three days, July 5, 6 and 7, 1932, in Dr. Kendall's laboratory at Northwestern University Medical School in Chicago. Assembled there to carry out the experiments were Dr. Kendall, Dr. Rosenow and myself. Owing to the novel and important character of the work, each of us verified at every step the results obtained.

The above mentioned reports serve to establish two important facts. First, that it is possible to cultivate viruses artificially, and, second, that viruses are definitely visible under the Rife Universal Microscope.

In our initial experiments we endeavor to cultivate bacteria in the filterable state. Certainly, the theoretical and practical importance of filterable organisms in theoretical and applied biology cannot be denied. However, later experiments led us to believe that the filterable form was a transitional state exhibited by bacteria when cultured under certain conditions. Actually it was found that this transitional form represented the virus phase of an organism in its life cycle.

During the incubation period of a pathogenic organism in a susceptible host, it is essential, if the disease germs are to be successful in producing the disease, that they upset the metabolic balance of the host and, particularly, the mineral salt balance of the cells. When this is accomplished to a certain degree the stage is set for a transition of the invading organisms into their primordial or virus state. It is the virus forms enacting upon the unbalanced constituents of the cells that produce the pathological changes associated with the disease. It must be remembered, before leaving this subject, that several phases in an organism's life cycle may exist.

The Rickettsia Bodies represent the primordial state of protozoa, just as the virus is the primordial form of bacteria. The staining reactions of the Rickettsia are similar to certain Treponemata, and their parasitic relations to certain insect hosts suggests relationships with the protozoa. Their refractoriness to artificial cultivation indicates their similarity to the virus form of bacterial.

We shall next consider the etiological relationships of Rickettsia to certain diseases.

We have confirmed the findings of Ricketts and Wilder which appear in a report published in the American Medical Association Journal, 1910 (Page 54). These workers observed the occurence of Rickettsia prowazeki in human typhus fever leisions. It has been shown that if lice infested with the Rickettsia bodies are ground up with salt solution when they are fully developed, they will induce Typhus fever in animals upon injection.

The similarity of the Rickettsia bodies associated with the Yellow fever group is astounding. The organism, Paraplasma faliaglum, is the parent phase of all the transitional forms in this group. The degree of cellular imbalance in the host determines the quality of the pathogenic changes. Severe imbalance results in a true Yellow fever, milder imbalance will give the indications of langue, and still milder imbalance will cause Phebotomus, or 3 day's fever (isoated, 1932).

Thus a new field is open to scientific investigators. The solution to the problem lies not in limitless classifications, but rather, in the fascinating study of the biochemical factors that cause these transitional forms known as virus and Rickettsia to be in the stage in which we find them.

Appendix G

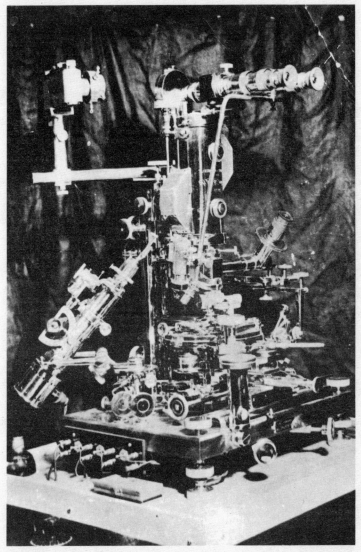

The Universal Microscope (1933)

Appendix H

RIFE RESEARCH LABORATORY   Sweence   · 80   1934

Operation and Investigation of Tumors In White Rats (3/14/4)

The tumor was located beneath the epithelial tissue covering the left side of the chest.

The duration of the operation was 55 minutes, during which time the animal was under ether anaesthesia.

The tumor weighed 60 g. and was of the Lipoma type. It was removed under sterile conditions and placed in glycerine immediately after the operation.

Three portions of tissue were removed from the center of the tumor. A tube of Sterile "K" media was inoculated with one portion. Another was sent to Dr. Ford for histological examination, and the third was ground in a sterile mortar containing sterile normal saline solution. The contents of the mortar was now passed thru a Berkfeld "W" filter and examined under 14,000 X magnification.

The fresh filtrate under the microscope revealed numerous ovoid granules, purplish red in color, and resembling the B.X. in morphology. The organisms are non-motile.

150

Appendix I

MILBANK JOHNSON, M. D.
PACIFIC MUTUAL LIFE BLDG.
LOS ANGELES, CALIFORNIA

April 30, 1934

My dear Doctor,

I am mailing you with this letter
a copy of the "Readers Digest" for May 1934.
There is an article entitled "Young Doctor
Heat" which I am very anxious to have you
read carefully. I have gotten a real idea
out of this which I want to discuss with you
next Saturday.

I wonder if your Ray could be the
short electro-magnetic wave referred to in
this article. Of course these people, having
no way to observe the effect on actual bacilli,
could not know the exact wave length or
oscillation on organisms.

This article seems to explain a great
deal to me that I did not know before and has
given me a great big idea which may be no good
but I do want to discuss it with you fully.

Can't you meet me about 11:30 in La Jolla
next Saturday. I want to show you the Library
Building and get your opinion of it before I say
anything to the people at the Scripps Clinic about it
as a place for our Clinic this Summer.

My biopsy forceps came this morning and I
also hope to bring down with me the penetration gages
which I think I told you about in my last letter.

Please try to meet me at the Casa de Manana
about 11:30 Saturday and we will have lunch together.

In haste,

Yours very sincerely,

Milbank Johnson

Dr. Royal R. Rife
2500 Chatsworth Blvd.
San Diego, California

600 BURLEIGH DRIVE
SAN RAFAEL HEIGHTS
PASADENA

151

Appendix J

8.1. The Technic of "BX" Inoculation

Our method of inoculation of experimental animals with "BX", the virus of cancer, is as follows:

The animal is first shaved and sterilized with alcohol and iodine solution at the point of inoculation and placed under partial anethesia. This avoids subjecting the animal to shock. An extra long, very small needle is used. The needle is filled with sterile petroleum jelly and a hypodermic is then filled with the inoculum and the needle placed on the syringe. The needle is inserted no less than 30 MM from the point of inoculation under the epidermis. The point of inoculation is in most cases the mammory gland for the reason that the "BX" involved was recovered from an unulcerated human breast mass.

In 3 to 4 days a legion appears in the thyroid area. The cause of this is unknown, but the legion recedes and heals over and a growth starts in the mammory gland of the experimental animal. These growths or tumors have exceeded the weight of the experimental animal in many cases. The tumor is surgically removed and the "BX" is again recovered in all cases.

An important factor and check is to make at least 10 transplants from the initial isolation of "BX". These transplants are made at 24 hour intervals into the original "K" media. This increases the virulence and speeds the growth of the tumor. With these experiments that have been repeated on over 100 experimental animals, we are convinced that this method definitely proves the virulence and pathology of "BX" virus.

If there are any workers interested in following this technic, we will furnish them with the formula of "K" media and all of the basic principles involved. However, it is beyond the scope of the average microscope to visualize these minute virus.

8.2. The Treatment of "BX" or Cancer

The actual cure of cancer in experimental animals occurs with the use of our frequency instrument. To attain these astounding results, a long and tedious process is started to determine the precise setting of the frequency instrument that is the mortal oscillatory rate of this virus. When the setting is found, it is repeated 10 consecutive times after the frequency instrument has been placed back to the same setting before a specific frequency is recorded. These results are observed under the high power of the universal microscope and when the mortal oscillatory rate is reached, the "BX" forms appear to "Blow Up" or disintegrate in the field. The inoculated animals are then subjected to the same frequency to determine if the effect is the same on the "BX" virus in the tissues of the experimental animals. The results are precisely identical with experimental animals as with the pure culture slides; these successful tests were conducted over 400 times with experimental animals before any attempt was made to use this frequency on human cases of carcinoma.

The first clinical work on cancer was completed under the supervision of Dr. Milbank Johnson M.D. which was set up under a special medical Research Committee of the University of Southern California. 16 cases were treated at the clinic for many types of malignancy. After 3 months, 14 of these so-called hopeless cases were signed off as clinically cured by the staff of five medical doctors and Dr. Alvin G. Foord, M.D. Pathologist for the group. The treatments consisted of 3 minutes duration using the frequency instrument which was set on the mortal oscillatory rate for "BX" or cancer (at 3 day intervals). It was found that the elapsed time between treatments attains better results than the cases treated daily. This give the lympatic system an opportunity to absorb and cast off a toxic condition which is produced by the devitalized dead particles of the

"BX" virus. No rise of body temperature was perceptable in any of these cases above normal during or after the frequency instrument treatment. No special diets were used in any of this clinical work, but we sincerely believe that a proper diet compiled for the individual would be of benefit.

The Determination and Diagnosis of Cancer

We can determine in over 90% of the cases of persons having carcinoma by the examination of a blood smear (with the technic heretofore explained) in 30 minutes. We have also found that in many types of epithelioma that the carcinoma tissue carries no conductivity with a pendulum galvonometer which enables us to outline and determine the location of a tumor without the use of X-Ray photographs. It has also been determined that any case of malignancy treated with either X-Ray or radium or other radio-active materials shows decided radio-activity and harmful tissue effects for many months after the treatments have been given. Destroyed tissue or tissue that has been harmed is a natural parasitic feast. We have also found that tumors treated with this method respond less readily to the treatment of our frequency instruments.

Appendix K

6.

<u>CHEMICAL RELATIVITY TO CARCINOMA</u>
<u>Coordinative Constituents</u>

(A) Dibenzanthracene as a carcinogenetic agent.

    1. Di-derivative of dis meaning separated by or doubling up.

    2. Benz -   (Benzene $C_6 H_6$)
          Benzol as a $C_6 H_6$ derivative $C_6 H_6$ nCH_2

    3. Anthracene - $C_{14} H_{10} = 3C_6 H_6 - C_4 H_8$ white solid Hydro-
carbon used in preparation of indigo and alizarin.

(B) Naphthalene ($6_{10} H_8$) almost same as $C_{14} H_{10}$ (moth balls).

Cancer Virus Characteristics

    1. Not destroyed by X-Ray, ultra violet ray or infra red ray.
    2. Thermal death point in 24 hours is 42 deg. C or 107. 6 deg. F.
    3. Sporogenous.
    4. Non liquifying (media).
    5. Non chromogenic and non aerobic.
    6. - (Cathode) polarization.
    7. Width of ovoid or micro-organism is 1/20 u.
    8. Length of ovoid micro-organism is 1/15 u.
    9. Flagellated and non parasitic.
  10. Highly motile and plastic.
  11. Highly pathogenic.
  12. Seen at 12 3/16° angle of refraction on universal microscope.
  13. Color of chemical refraction is purple red, which results from
the coordinative constituents reacting upon the degree of light
frequency applied.

Appendix L

NORTHWESTERN UNIVERSITY MEDICAL SCHOOL
303 EAST CHICAGO AVENUE
CHICAGO, ILLINOIS

Department of Research Bacteriology
Ward Memorial Building

September 20, 1934

Dear Mrs. Bridges:

My wife and I were unfortunately not able to pay our respects to you before we left California.and this is both an apology and also a renewed expression of our pleasure in being invited to your very beautiful party. We do hope we shall be fortunate enough to be in California again so we may call upon you.

Our trip home was without incident: it was hot the first day, but we succeeded in getting a place in an air conditioned car, and the remainder of the journey was very comfortable. It was quite cool when we landed in Chicago, and it has been comfortable ever since. We have been away for two and one half months, so everything was strange, especially the bustle and confusion of a large city which we both detest. We believe the ideal arrangement would be to live in LaJolla ten months of the year, and in Old Mexico the remainder. Our visit to Mexico was one of the outstanding episodes of our lives, and we really became very fond of the country, especially of the Hacienda in the State of Durango where we spent five weeks. Another year we hope to know enough Spanish to carry on a conversation:at present we are limited to bare necessities:eating, travelling (provided there are no emergencies which would call for words not in our vocabulary) and doing the very ordinary things of life. My wife has promised to study the language this winter, and I have already spent some three months learning the rudiments, so it may be that another year we may really converse with the Spanish people in their own tongue, a most desirable accomplishment.

This after noon I have a meeting with Mr. Hardin, President of the Board of Trustees of the University:he is much interested in Roy and his splendid work, and I shall be asked to tell what I saw during my very brief visit to California. Mr. Hardin, unlike many persons, is very friendly, and will take the proper view point of the work:that it is experimental so far, done with no rules of the game to go by, and with a machine that is designed for small output, and therefore, not capable of showing its full worth. I understand there is to be a new machine, embodying the facts learned from the old one, and built along more lusty lines so its output will be more nearly equal to the demands which should be put upon it. I have written to Dr. Johnson telling him about the one case I can talk intelligently about:Tom KHight. Roy (Rife) will tell you about Tom:he seems to me to be the most important case of the entire series because his tumor was on the cheek, where it could be seen, watched and measured from the start to the finish. This I have done, reciting the actual measurements, and details of treatment and of pathological examination.

I do hope you will overlook the use of the typewriter:my handwriting is so very bad no one, including myself can read it. Hence I substitute impoliteness for illegibility.

My wife unites with me in warmest regards,

Ever sincerely yours,

155

Appendix M

MILBANK JOHNSON, M.D.
PACIFIC MUTUAL LIFE BLDG.
LOS ANGELES, CALIFORNIA

March 11, 1935

My dear Dr. Rife,

Inclosed you will find a letter which I have just received from the International Cancer Research Foundation.

In order that I may most effectively comply with their request, will you send me some pictures taken of the interior of your laboratory, also a picture of the big microscope. Also, will you answer as many of their questions as you see fit as they are naturally interested in knowing as much as possible about your accomplishments.

Please do this as soon as you can because I want to get these people back there started as soon as possible. Will you return their letter for my files.

Yours very sincerely,

[signature: Milbank Johnson]

Dr. Royal R. Rife
2500 Chatsworth Blvd.
San Diego, Calif.

600 BURLEIGH DRIVE
SAN RAFAEL HEIGHTS
PASADENA

Appendix N

MILBANK JOHNSON, M.D.
PACIFIC MUTUAL LIFE BLDG.
LOS ANGELES, CALIFORNIA

May 9, 1935

My dear Doctor,

As Mrs. Johnson and I are coming down to San Diego Saturday, I would like, with your permission, to have Charles bring Mrs. Young along with him so that she can have another Ray treatment.

She is very much improved. All of the small seed glands in both sides of the neck have disappeared. This morning when I examined her there was only one gland on the right side, just above the clavicle, much smaller than originally and less painful. The three palpable glands on the left side were smaller than when examined on April 29 and not painful. I think, however, to make assurance doubly sure that we will give her another shot Saturday before noon if it is agreeable to you. If not, please wire me and I will not bring her down.

Yours very sincerely,

Milbank Johnson

She was cured of T.B.
"Dr. Couvivns" brothers wife"

Dr. Royal R. Rife
2500 Chatsworth Blvd.
San Diego, Calif.

P.S. Unless I hear from you to the contrary I will bring Mrs. Young down.

600 BURLEIGH DRIVE
SAN RAFAEL HEIGHTS
PASADENA

157

Appendix O

If it would not be asking too much, you might
bring your petrographic and that slide of the
onion skin which would give them some idea of
the action of the variable monochromatic beam.

A few days ago I received a report from
Dr. Foord of the postmortem of a guinea pig which
he inoculated from some of the glands taken in the
last operation from Mrs. Young, Charles' wife. It
showed a distinct, but not bad, tubercular infection
in the glands of the guinea pig, a few living
tubercular bacilli. He said they were rather long
and a few of them were beaded. He pronounced the
diagnosis postively tuberculosis.

Now, it has occurred to me, that if he
found no living tubercular bacilli, or anything that
looks like them, in the sections of the glands *of Mrs. Young*
themselves, or in a stained slide made from a caseous
material taken therefrom, I am inclined to believe
that in these old tubercular lesions that probably
were so "Much" granules which, as we know, will not
develop in artificial culture, nor do they show in
cold abscesses very often, but, still, if injected
into guinea pigs produce tubercle bacilli: maybe
these Much glands are another form of the same ~~thing~~ *T.B.*
corresponding to our filter passing form and we will
have to get an M. O. R. for them so as to destroy
them at the same time that we do the rod form of
tuberculosis.

I am quite satisfied that we will run no
danger in radiating with the Rife Ray moderate cases
of tuberculosis. In discussing the matter with
Dr. Dock, he advises by all means to take a chance
and any reaction that we might obtain can probably be
handled symptomatically. It will require a great deal
of work to find an M. O. R. for these Much granules.
You will find them described on page 224 of Kendall's
Bacteriology, 2nd Edition. They are probably described
in all of his editions but maybe not on the same page.

Appendix P

MILBANK JOHNSON, M. D.
PACIFIC MUTUAL LIFE BLDG.
LOS ANGELES, CALIFORNIA

October 8, 1935

My dear Dr. Rife,

We are about ready to begin our clinical work with the new Rife Ray Machine which seems to be a great success. It has much greater power and penetration than the original which we used last summer.

There are many improvements in this machine which are possible through the great improvements made in radio technique. There is not a moving part, for example, in our new machine and hence we expect it to have a much longer life with harder usage.

We believe it wise to protect the members of the Committee and the physicians from suits for damages. Your Chairman, therefore, has had prepared by experienced lawyers two forms of release which I am submitting to you for your suggestions or approval. Kindly read them over very carefully. Consult any attorney you please if you so desire, and return them to me as promptly as possible as we are about ready to start.

We have tested the machine out very thoroughly both on animals and on cultures, and so far as we can see, it leaves nothing to be desired.

Hoping that you will examine and return the releases to me with your comments as quickly as possible, I am

Yours very sincerely,

Milbank Johnson Chairman

Special Medical Research Committee of
the University of Southern California

Dr. Royal Raymond Rife
2500 Chatsworth Boulevard
San Diego, California

800 BURLEIGH DRIVE
SAN RAFAEL HEIGHTS
PASADENA

Appendix Q

MILBANK JOHNSON, M. D.
PACIFIC MUTUAL LIFE BLDG.
LOS ANGELES, CALIFORNIA

December 19, 1935

My dear Dr. Rife,

A meeting of the Special Medical Research Committee of the University of Southern California will be held Thursday, December 26 at 12:15 P.M. in Room 2 of the California Club.

As Dr. George Dock, a member of our Committee, is leaving on January 2 for a trip around the World and will not return for several months, I am anxious to have this meeting before he leaves as there are many things of importance to be considered. We have much to report and are very anxious to receive your advice on some questions of vital importance to the work.

I trust you will make a special effort to attend. I have tried to trouble the members of the Committee as little as possible with meetings, but it becomes absolutely necessary now that we should meet and decide some vital points.

You might call Dr. Burger and see if you can't arrange to come up together as you did last time. Also, it will keep him from forgetting it and insure his being here if you bring him.

Please let me hear from you as to whether or not you can be present at this meeting.

Wishing you and Mrs. Rife a Merry Christmas and a Happy New Year, I am

Yours very sincerely,

Milbank Johnson, Chairman
Special Medical Research Committee
University of Southern California

Dr. R. R. Rife
2500 Chatsworth Blvd.
San Diego, California

600 BURLEIGH DRIVE
SAN RAFAEL HEIGHTS
PASADENA

160

Appendix R

MILBANK JOHNSON, M. D.
~~RADIO CONTINENTAL BUILDING~~
LOS ANGELES, CALIFORNIA
Subway Terminal Building

January 4, 1937

My dear Roy:

I wrote you sometime ago that I had the p.H. machine for you, and all it needs now is some means of transportation to San Diego. I also have the full instruction book that goes with it. I had hoped before this that we would be coming down, but we have moved, having disposed of Belbank, and hence have been unable to get away. Our new address is 710 Pinehurst Drive, Pasadena, near the Huntington Hotel.

I have had several conversations with Dr. Charles Martin, former Dean of McGill University in Montreal, who has been out here for a few days. I tried my best to get him down to San Diego, but he simply could not get the time to go. However, I had several interviews with him and Sir Montague Allen and Dr. Dook. Between us, we succeeded in selling him the idea that it would be a good thing for Dr. Gruner to be sent out here by McGill. Dr. Martin is still on the Board of Governors of the University and he has undertaken to do his very best to get McGill to send us Dr. Gruner, McGill paying Dr. Gruner's salary and expenses. Dr. Martin will arrive back in Montreal by the first of February when, he says, we may expect to hear definite developments on this subject. Sir Montague feels pretty certain that Dr. Gruner will be sent.

There are so many things that I would like to discuss with you, and also I want you to get the p.H. machine down to the laboratory, so I wish you could come up here some day soon. Let me know before you get here so we can start the new year pulling together for our common goal, namely, success.

Mrs. Johnson joins me in wishing you and Mrs. Rife a happy and prosperous New Year.

Yours very sincerely,

MILBANK JOHNSON

P. S. Please let me know when you can come up.

600 BURLEIGH DRIVE
SAN RAFAEL HEIGHTS
PASADENA

161

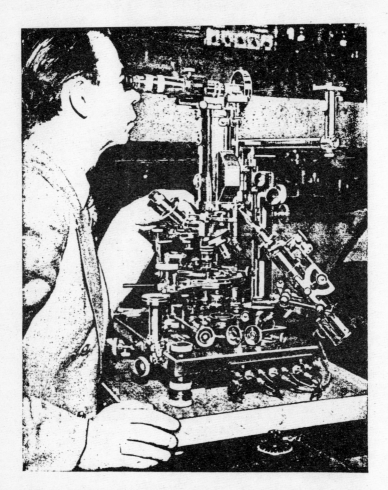

Giant Microscope Explores New Worlds

REPORTED to be so powerful that it reveals disease organisms never seen before, the giant microscope pictured above has just been completed by Royal R. Rife, of San Diego, Calif., whose home-built instruments have long been ranked among the finest in the world. To eliminate distortion, the image produced by the new two-foot-tall apparatus does not pass through the usual air-filled tube, but along an optical path of quartz blocks and prisms. Weighing 200 pounds, the microscope has 5,682 parts.

OCTOBER, 1940

Appendix T

RES 4491 SANTA CRUZ

CHARLES F. TULLY, D. D. S.
PRACTICE LIMITED TO
SURGERY AND DENTURES
OFFICE: 2054 LOGAN AVENUE
SAN DIEGO, CALIFORNIA

June 1, 1954

It is with difficulty that I attempt to respond to your request for data on the Frequency Instrument treatments since I am moving and am very busy.

My knowledge of the Frequency Instrument treatment extends over a number of years, although my personal use of the Frequency Instrument has been in the last few years. My first definite investigation was in that of my own case of prostatitis, I tried medicines. A qualified urologist gave me gantrisin, penicillin, aureomycin, chloromycitin terramycin, with various results but the drugs did not do the job. The Frequency Instrument cured my case quickly. I then used the Frequency Instrument on a friend of mine who was being rushed to the hospital for a prostrate operation. He is perfectly well today without any operation or further medical aid.

I had a case of butterfly lupus sent to me by a doctor friend, and though it had been treated extensively and by specialists, the condition was large and in progression. After three months treatment with the Frequency Instrument, the butterfly lupus disappeared. Another cancer (carcinoma) case was submitted to me for treatment with the Frequency Instrument by an M.D. friend of mine. He had an impossible condition but the Frequency Instrument dried it up in six weeks.

I have found the Frequency Instrument very effective after surgery. I use it alone instead of antibiotics and have not had a case of infection. I have cured extremely bad cases of trench mouth and pyorrea in a few treatments with the Frequency Instrument.

In conclusion I must state that I feel that the Frequency Instrument is worthy of further research and that subsequent investigation and use will be of great benefit to all mankind.

Most sincerely yours,

Charles F. Tully

Charles F. Tully

163

Appendix U

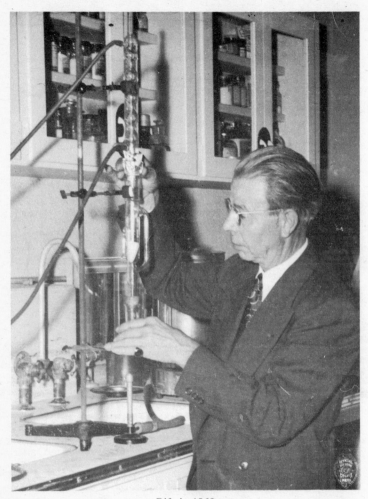

Rife in 1960

Appendix V

677 S. Burlington Ave.
Los Angeles, Calif., 90057
January 7, 1965.

To Whom It May Concern:

In the spring of 1960 I contacted a staph. Aureus infection while an interne at St. Alexis Hospital in Cleveland, Ohio. This was a plague in this hospital as is still prevalent in most U.S. hospitals..difficult to control.

The infection started with a threat culture which was suppressed with anti-biotics. Soon after,I with about 6 others,became a victim of this anti-biotic resistant infection which became systemic and chronic.

It was three years of suffering until I came across the Frequency Instrument which gave me immediate relief and control so that I was then on the road for a"CURE."I used the Model SQ2, Serial No. 20, RVM 12 as manufactured by the Rife Virus Microscope Institute of San Diego, California.

This systemic infection disappeared after five days of intensive treatment. Indeed it was a great relief to get rid of the extensive cellulitis for the length of the left lower leg with edema of the foot and ankle with discoloration and multiple boils and carbuncles reappearing which required two hospitalizations and continuous treatment for three years. Indeed I just about gave up.

Logically no research or interest in any new field especially in the healing arts and science should be suppressed. It has been stated, again and again, that one is a martyr to his profession. Such I find true in any research adventure. It takes a lot of courage, time, money and hard work to find new methods.

I am of the opinion and belief that if I had not had the treament on the Frequency Instrument above that I would not be able to get rid of this incurable staph. aureus which anti-biotics could not suppress.

It left me with a deformed right hand and wrist along with the arm in which the distal end of the radial bone shows permanent distorted damage on x-ray study and observation which has reduced the efficiency of the use of this hand and arm about Fifty per-cent.

I am grateful to have had the privilege of the use of this instrument which appears as a specific for certain virus'.

I am for any and all freedom of research where life, health and happiness can be improved.

Yours very truly,

George Chromiak, Jr., M.D.
Phone: Area Code 213, 483-7448

Affidavit
To Whom It May Concern:
Sworn and subscribed before me.................... a Notary public this 7th Day of Januray 1965 in Los Angeles, California.

Notary Public

M. Commission Expires Nov 23, 1968

Appendix W

AFFIDAVIT OF MRS. BLANCHE H. JONES OF 1840
4th Avenue, Apt. 28, SAN DIEGO, CALIFORNIA
CURE FROM CANCER BY THE RIFE
FREQUENCY INSTRUMENT AFTER 12 YEARS.

I, Blanche H. Jones, as Counsel in Pro Per,
do hereby certify that in April 1956 I was diagnosed as having
cancer and was operated on by five M.D.s at the San Diego County
Hospital and one breast was removed and it was reported that the
cancer was still in my body and pus drainage was severe. In May 1956
I was given treatments by the Rife Frequency Instrument by Dr. James
B. Couche,M.D. which stopped the flow of pus and cured my sarcoma
as diagnosed by Dr. Worthylake,M.D. and others by biopsy.

The Frequency Instrument was such a wonderful
Godsend. It saved my life! It has been twelve years now since it
cured my cancer and I give this statement under penalty of perjury
as being true and correct.

STATE OF CALIFORNIA)
                    (ss
COUNTY OF SAN DIEGO)

Subscribed and Sworn to
before me this 16th day
of January, 1968

LUCILLE GROTZ
COUNTY OF SAN DIEGO
NOTARY PUBLIC

ATTEST my hand this 16th day of
January, 1968

MRS. BLANCHE H. JONES in pro per

166

Appendix X

Devised & Compiled by R. R. Rife 1920 to 1953

Copyright 1953 - by Allied Industries

RESEARCH SUMMARY OF BACTERIA AND VIRUS CHARACTERISTICS

Micro-Organism	Motile	Flagellated	Polarity Anode +	Polarity Cathode −	Length u	Width u	Death Pt. Milli-amps D.C.	Thermal Death Pt. °C.	Thermal death Pt. (24 hrs.) °C.	Death by X-Ray	Death by infra-red Violet	Death by Ultra Violet	Dye	Aerobic	Acid Resisting (to dye)
Syphilis	yes	no		X	3.5-16.5	.33-.5	80	39.5	103.1	slight	no	no	Silver Nitrate	yes	no
Tuberculosis	no	no	X		1.5-3.3	.8	168	42.5	107.8	no	slight	no	Gentian Violet	yes	yes
Gonorrhea	no	no	X		1.6	.8	8.3	39	102.2	no	helps growth	slight	Carmine	yes	no
Leprosy	no	no	X		1.4-3.3	2-3.5	58	42	105.8	slight	no	no	Carmine	either	yes
Actinomycosis	no	no		X	Long	.3-.5	12.2	40	104	slight	no	no	Bismark Brown	either	no
Typhoid	yes	yes		X	1.3-2.4	.5-.8	28	39.5	103.1	no	no	no	Gentian Violet	either	no
Catarrhal Inflammation	no	no	X		12.0	1.0	76	47	116.6	no	no	no	Gishma	either	no
Bacillus Coli	yes	yes	X		1.3	.4-.7	7	45	113	no	slight	no	Gentian Violet	either	no
Bubonic Plague	no	no	X		1.5-2	.5-.75	140	48	118.4	no	no	no	Gentian Violet	either	no
Tetanus	no	no		X	2.4	.3-.5	64	51.5	132.9	slight	slight	slight	Silver Nitrate	either	slight
Diptheria	no	no		X	1.5-6.5	.3-.8	175	45	113	slight	no	no	Hematoxyline	yes	no
Symptomatic Anthrax	yes	yes			3.5	.6-.8	71	49.5	120.4	no	slight	no	Gentian Violet	no	yes
Anthrax	no	no		X	5.2	1-1.25	75	45	113	no	no	no	Gentian Violet	either	no
Pneumonia	no	no		X	2-5 Diam		12	47	116.6	no	no	no	Hematoxyline	either	no
Spinal Meningitis	no	no		X	2-.6 Diam		110	48	118.4	no	no	slight	Silver Nitrate	either	no
Glanders	no	no	X		1.5-3	.25-.4	95	50.6	123.08	no	no	no	Bismark Brown	either	no
Cholera	yes	yes	X		.8-2.5	1-.04	74	43	109.4	no	no	slight	Hematoxyline	either	no
Typhus	yes	yes		−	.5	.2	120	50	122	no	no	slight	Bismark Brown	yes	no
Influenza	no	no		X	1-2	.25	89	42	105.8	no	no	slight	Silver Nitrate	yes	no
Contagious Conjunctivitis	no	no	X		7 Diam		89	40°	104	no	no	no	Silver Nitrate	either	no
Staphlococcus	no	no		X	.4-1 Diam.		120	50	122	no	no	no	Hematoxyline	either	no
Streptococcus	no	no		X											
												Universal Microscope Angle of color of refraction chemical for light refraction		
Cancer Virus	yes	yes		X	1/16	1/20	175	42°C	107.6	no	no	no	−12.3/10°	no	no
Typhoid Virus	yes	yes	X		1/8	1/11	128	41	105.8	no	no	no	+4.8°	yes	no
B. Coli Virus	yes	yes	X		1/8	1/10	86	43	109.4	no	no	no	+7°	yes	no
Polio Virus	yes	yes		X	1/10	1/14							+8.5°	yes	no
Herpes Virus	no	no		−	1/11	1/15							+14°	no	no

Beware of Exploiters!

Over the years since this book was first published, a number of garage engineers, marketing hustlers and scam artists, along with well-meaning but misleading alternative cancer therapy advocates, have offered various "black box" devices as real or "improved" Rife instruments. These range in price from $300 to $3000 or more. I warn the interested reader of this book to be careful in purchasing any such instrument or even taking and especially paying for a "treatment" from someone who thinks they own a "Rife" device.

For anyone actually diagnosed with cancer, this warning is all the more serious. Unless you have investigated the results obtained with a given "Rife" instrument and found it to have been successful with a significant number of real people with cancer, with whom you have personally spoken, don't waste your time or money. There are better alternative cancer therapies available with better track records than most of the machines being marketed as "Rife" devices at the current time.

Still, "resonance healing" is coming along at an accelerating pace and *there are* Rife instruments which, combined with dedicated practitioners and carefully developed protocols, are accomplishing stunning healing. The only impediment to their open testing and widespread use is the prevailing political and legal climate!

Those interested in working toward changing that climate may contact me at the address below, but do bring something to the table, not "I want to help but don't know how." This invitation does not include cancer patients seeking personal advice on any specific "Rife" device. Remember, most are junk even if the promotional advertisements are slick and sound wonderful (the marketing hustlers are alive and well). If you expect a reply (I do not promise one), do include a self-addressed, stamped envelope.

Barry Lynes
P. O. Box 12183
Palm Desert, CA
USA 92255